A Practical Guide to

Botulinum Toxin Procedures

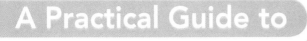
A Practical Guide to

Botulinum Toxin Procedures

Series Editor

Rebecca Small, M.D., F.A.A.F.P.

Assistant Clinical Professor,
Family and Community Medicine,
University of California, San Francisco, CA

Director, Medical Aesthetics Training,
Natividad Medical Center,
Family Medicine Residency Program—UCSF Affiliate,
Salinas, CA

Private Practice,
Capitola, CA

Associate Editor

Dalano Hoang, D.C.

Clinic Director,
Monterey Bay Laser Aesthetics,
Capitola, CA

 Wolters Kluwer | Lippincott Williams & Wilkins
Health

Philadelphia • Baltimore • New York • London
Buenos Aires • Hong Kong • Sydney • Tokyo

Acquisitions Editor: Sonya Seigafuse
Product Manager: Kerry Barrett
Production Manager: Bridgett Dougherty
Senior Manufacturing Manager: Benjamin Rivera
Marketing Manager: Kim Schonberger
Creative Director: Doug Smock
Production Service: Aptara, Inc.

Printed in The United States of America

Library of Congress Cataloging-in-Publication Data
Small, Rebecca.
 A practical guide to botulinum toxin procedures / Rebecca Small ;
associate editor, Dalano Hoang.
   p. cm.
 Includes bibliographical references and index.
 ISBN-13: 978-1-60913-147-0 (alk. paper)
 ISBN-10: 1-60913-147-9 (alk. paper)
 1. Botulinum toxin–Therapeutic use. 2. Injections, Intradermal.
I. Hoang, Dalano. II. Title.
 [DNLM: 1. Botulinum Toxins–therapeutic use–Handbooks. 2. Cosmetic
Techniques–Handbooks. 3. Injections, Intradermal–methods–Handbooks.
QV 39]
 RL120.B66S63 2012
 615′.778–dc23

                                                2011015537

Care has been taken to confirm the accuracy of the information presented and to describe generally accepted practices. However, the authors, editors, and publisher are not responsible for errors or omissions or for any consequences from application of the information in this book and make no warranty, expressed or implied, with respect to the currency, completeness, or accuracy of the contents of the publication. Application of the information in a particular situation remains the professional responsibility of the practitioner.

The authors, editors, and publisher have exerted every effort to ensure that drug selection and dosage set forth in this text are in accordance with current recommendations and practice at the time of publication. However, in view of ongoing research, changes in government regulations, and the constant flow of information relating to drug therapy and drug reactions, the reader is urged to check the package insert for each drug for any change in indications and dosage and for added warnings and precautions. This is particularly important when the recommended agent is a new or infrequently employed drug.

Some drugs and medical devices presented in the publication have Food and Drug Administration (FDA) clearance for limited use in restricted research settings. It is the responsibility of the health care providers to ascertain the FDA status of each drug or device planned for use in their clinical practice.

To purchase additional copies of this book, call our customer service department at (800) 638-3030 or fax orders to (301) 223-2320. International customers should call (301) 223-2300.

Visit Lippincott Williams & Wilkins on the Internet: at LWW.com. Lippincott Williams & Wilkins customer service representatives are available from 8:30 am to 6 pm, EST.

16

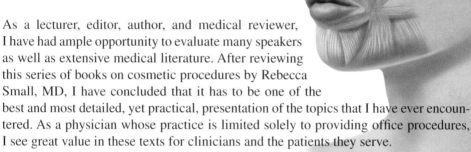

Foreword

As a lecturer, editor, author, and medical reviewer, I have had ample opportunity to evaluate many speakers as well as extensive medical literature. After reviewing this series of books on cosmetic procedures by Rebecca Small, MD, I have concluded that it has to be one of the best and most detailed, yet practical, presentation of the topics that I have ever encountered. As a physician whose practice is limited solely to providing office procedures, I see great value in these texts for clinicians and the patients they serve.

The goal of medical care is to make patients feel better and to help them experience an improved quality of life that extends for an optimal, productive period. Interventions may be directed at the emotional/psychiatric, medical/physical, or self-image areas.

For many physicians, performing medical procedures provides excitement in the practice of medicine. The ability to see what has been accomplished in a concrete way provides the positive feedback we all seek in providing care. Sometimes, it involves removing a tumor. At other times, it may be performing a screening procedure to be sure no disease is present. Maybe it is making patients feel better about their appearance. For whatever reason, the "hands on" practice of medicine is more rewarding for some practitioners.

In the late 1980s and early 1990s, there was resurgence in the interest of performing procedures in primary care. It did not involve hospital procedures but rather those that could be performed in the office. Coincidentally, patients also became interested in less invasive procedures such as laparoscopic cholecystectomy, endometrial ablation, and more. The desire for plastic surgery "extreme makeovers" waned, as technology was developed to provide a gentle, more kind approach to "rejuvenation." Baby boomers were increasing in numbers and wanted to maintain their youthful appearance. This not only improved self-image but it also helped when competing with a younger generation both socially and in the workplace.

These forces then of technological advances, provider interest, and patient desires have led to a huge increase in and demand for "minimally invasive procedures" that has extended to all of medicine. Plastic surgery and aesthetic procedures have indeed been affected by this movement. There have been many new procedures developed in just the last 10–15 years along with constant updates and improvements. As patient demand has soared for these new treatments, physicians have found that there is a whole new world of procedures they need to incorporate into their practice if they are going to provide the latest in aesthetic services.

Rebecca Small, MD, the editor and author of this series of books on cosmetic procedures, has been at the forefront of the aesthetic procedures movement. She has written extensively and conducted numerous workshops to help others learn the latest techniques. She has the practical experience to know just what the physician needs to develop a practice and provides "the latest and the best" in these books. Using her knowledge of the field, she has selected the topics wisely to include

- A Practical Guide to: Botulinum Toxin Procedures
- A Practical Guide to: Dermal Filler Procedures
- A Practical Guide to: Skin Care Procedures and Products
- A Practical Guide to: Cosmetic Laser Procedures

Dr. Small does not just provide a cursory, quick review of these subjects. Rather, they are an in-depth practical guide to performing these procedures. The emphasis here should be on "practical" and "in depth." There is no extra esoteric waste of words, yet every procedure is explained in a clear, concise, useful format that allows practitioners of all levels of experience to learn and gain from reading these texts.

The basic outline of these books consists of the pertinent anatomy, the specific indications and contraindications, specific how to diagram and explanations on performing the procedures, complications and how to deal with them, tables with comparisons and amounts of materials needed, before and after patient instructions as well as consent forms (an immense time-saving feature), sample procedure notes, and a list of supply sources. An extensive updated bibliography is provided in each text for further reading. Photos are abundant depicting the performance of the procedures as well as before and after results. These comprehensive texts are clearly written for the practitioner who wants to "learn everything" about the topics covered. Patients definitely desire these procedures, and Dr. Small has provided the information to meet the physician demand to learn them.

For those interested in aesthetic procedures, these books will be a godsend. Even for those not so interested in performing the procedures described, the reading is easy and interesting and will update the reader on what is currently available so they might better advise their patients.

Dr. Small has truly written a one-of-a-kind series of books on Cosmetic Procedures. It is my prediction that it will be received very well and be most appreciated by all who make use of it.

John L. Pfenninger, MD, FAAFP
Founder and President, The Medical Procedures Center
PC Founder and Senior Consultant, The National Procedures Institute
Clinical Professor of Family Medicine, Michigan State College
of Human Medicine

Preface

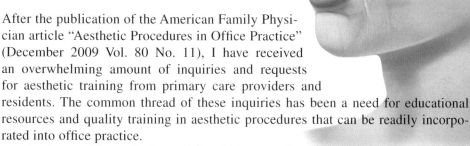

After the publication of the American Family Physician article "Aesthetic Procedures in Office Practice" (December 2009 Vol. 80 No. 11), I have received an overwhelming amount of inquiries and requests for aesthetic training from primary care providers and residents. The common thread of these inquiries has been a need for educational resources and quality training in aesthetic procedures that can be readily incorporated into office practice.

As the trend in aesthetic medicine shifts away from surgical procedures that can radically alter appearance, toward procedures that have minimal recovery time and offer more subtle enhancements, the number of minimally invasive aesthetic procedures performed continues to increase. These procedures, which include botulinum toxin and dermal filler injections, lasers and light-based technologies, and exfoliation treatments, have become the primary modalities for treatment of facial aging and skin rejuvenation. This aesthetic procedures series is designed to be a truly practical guide for physicians, physician assistants, nurse practitioners, residents in training, and other health care providers interested in aesthetics. It is not comprehensive but is inclusive of current minimally invasive aesthetic procedures that can be readily incorporated into office practice, which directly benefit our patients and achieve good outcomes with a low incidence of side effects.

This botulinum toxin injection book is the first in the aesthetic practical guide series and is intended for both novice practitioners learning a new aesthetic procedure, and for more seasoned practitioners seeking advanced procedures. Providers-in-training and teachers can benefit from the step-by-step approach and the online videos of each procedure performed by the author. Also included are suggestions for management of the most commonly encountered issues seen in follow-up visits. Seasoned practitioners may appreciate the concise summary of each procedure's complications and up-to-date suggestions for management, combining aesthetic treatments to maximize outcomes, current product developments, and reimbursement recommendations.

The Introduction and Foundation Concepts section in this book, provides basic aesthetic medicine concepts essential to successfully performing aesthetic procedures. Each chapter is dedicated to a single botulinum toxin procedure with all relevant anatomy reviewed, including the target muscles and their functions, as well as the muscles to be avoided. Injection points and the injection *safety zones* are highlighted to help the providers perform the procedures more effectively and minimize complications. The first three chapters, which cover treatment in the upper third of the face for frown lines, horizontal forehead lines, and crow's feet, are ideal for providers getting started with cosmetic botulinum toxin treatments. The remaining chapters of the book cover more advanced cosmetic treatments in the lower face, neck, and axillary hyperhidrosis.

This book is intended to serve as a guide and not a replacement for experience. When learning aesthetic procedural skills, preceptorship with a skilled provider or a formal training course is recommended to minimize undesired outcomes. When getting started with these procedures, providers may consider performing initial treatments on staff and family to get feedback and closely observe the effects of botulinum toxin. Also consider receiving a treatment to gain personal knowledge about botulinum toxin procedures.

Acknowledgments

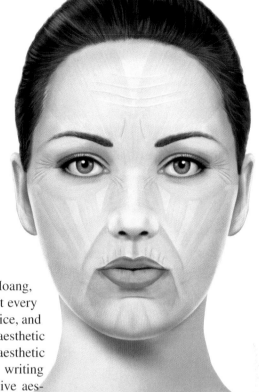

I have profound gratitude and respect for Dr. Dalano Hoang, my associate editor and husband. He has been with me at every step of the way as the clinic director of our aesthetic practice, and much more. Although he personally does not perform aesthetic procedures, his knowledge of the multiple aspects of aesthetic medicine is extensive and invaluable. His clear, concise writing style combined with my knowledge of minimally invasive aesthetic procedures yielded this straightforward procedure book.

A special thanks to Drs. John L. Pfenninger and E. J. Mayeaux, who have inspired and supported me, and taught me much about educating and writing.

The University of California, San Francisco and the Natividad Medical Center family medicine residents deserve special recognition. Their interest and enthusiasm for aesthetic procedures led me to develop the first family medicine aesthetics training curriculum in 2008. Special recognition is also due to the primary-care providers who participated in my aesthetic courses at the American Academy of Family Physicians' national conferences over the years. Their questions and input further solidified the need for this practical guide series.

I am indebted to my Capitola office staff for their ongoing logistical and administrative support, which made it possible to write this series.

Special acknowledgments are due to those at Wolters Kluwer Health, who made this book series possible, in particular, Kerry Barrett, Sonya Seigafuse, Freddie Patane, Brett MacNaughton, and Doug Smock. It has been a pleasure working with Liana Bauman, the gifted artist who created all of the illustrations for these books.

Finally, I would like to dedicate this book to my 5-year-old son, Kaidan Hoang, for the unending hugs and kisses that greeted me no matter how late I got home from working on this project.

Contents

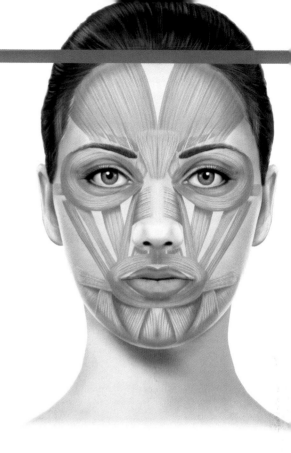

   A video clip for every procedure can be found on the book's website.

Anatomy

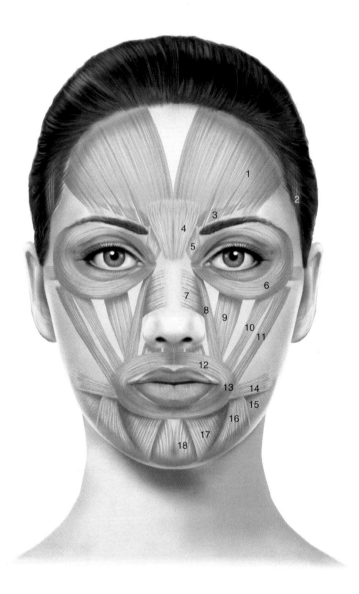

1. Frontalis m.
2. Temporalis m.
3. Corrugator supercilii m.
4. Procerus m.
5. Depressor supercilii m.
6. Orbicularis oculi m.
7. Nasalis m.
8. Levator labii superioris alaeque nasi m.
9. Levator labii superioris m.
10. Zygomaticus minor m.
11. Zygomaticus major m.
12. Orbicularis oris m.
13. Modeolus
14. Risorius m.
15. Platysma m.
16. Depressor anguli oris m.
17. Depressor labii inferioris m.
18. Mentalis m.

FIGURE 1 ● Musculature of the face–anterior-posterior. Copyright R. Small, MD.

1

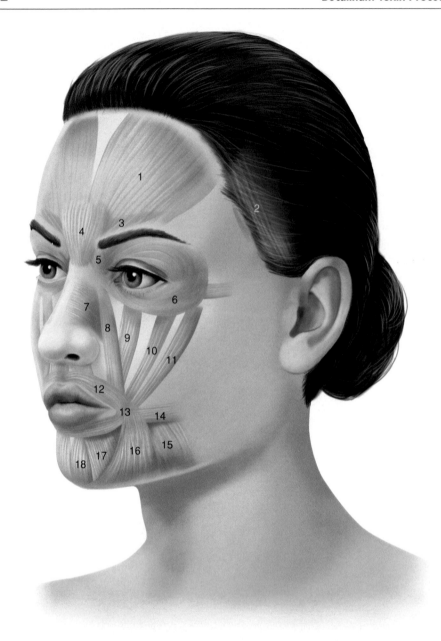

1. Frontalis m.
2. Temporalis m.
3. Corrugator supercilii m.
4. Procerus m.
5. Depressor supercilii m.
6. Orbicularis oculi m.
7. Nasalis m.
8. Levator labii superioris alaeque nasi m.
9. Levator labii superioris m.
10. Zygomaticus minor m.
11. Zygomaticus major m.
12. Orbicularis oris m.
13. Modeolus
14. Risorius m.
15. Platysma m.
16. Depressor anguli oris m.
17. Depressor labii inferioris m.
18. Mentalis m.

FIGURE 2 ● Musculature of the face–oblique. Copyright R. Small, MD.

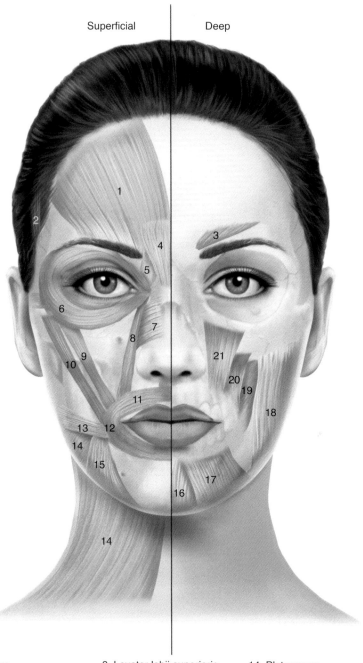

Superficial | Deep

FIGURE 3 ● Superficial and deep musculature of the face. Copyright R. Small, MD.

1. Frontalis m.
2. Temporalis m.
3. Corrugator supercilii m.
4. Procerus m.
5. Depressor supercilii m.
6. Orbicularis oculi m.
7. Nasalis m.

8. Levator labii superioris
   alaeque nasi m.
9. Zygomaticus minor m.
10. Zygomaticus major m.
11. Orbicularis oris m.
12. Modeulus
13. Risorius m.

14. Platysma m.
15. Depressor anguli oris m.
16. Mentalis m.
17. Depressor labii inferioris m.
18. Masseter m.
19. Buccinator m.
20. Levator anguli oris m.
21. Levator labii superioris m.

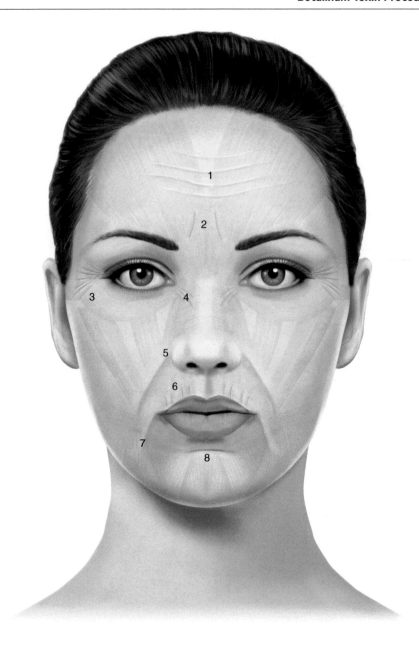

1. Horizontal forehead lines
   (Frontalis m.)
2. Frown lines
   (Glabellar complex m.)
3. Crow's feet
   (Orbicularis oculi m.)
4. Bunny lines
   (Nasalis m.)
5. Nasolabial folds
   (Levator labii superioris alaeque nasi m.)
6. Radial lip lines
   (Orbicularis oris m.)
7. Marionette lines
   (Depressor anguli oris m.)
8. Chin line
   (Mentalis m.)

FIGURE 4 ● Wrinkles and folds of the face–anterior-posterior (contributing muscle).
Copyright R. Small, MD.

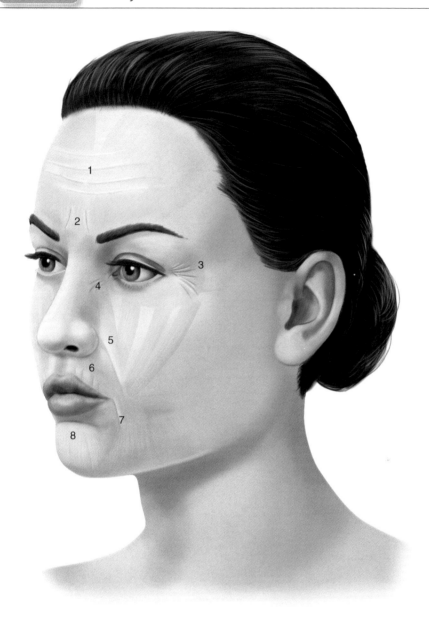

1. Horizontal forehead lines
   (Frontalis m.)
2. Frown lines
   (Glabellar complex m.)
3. Crow's feet
   (Orbicularis oculi m.)
4. Bunny lines
   (Nasalis m.)
5. Nasolabial folds
   (Levator labii superioris alequae nasi m.)
6. Radial lip lines
   (Orbicularis oris m.)
7. Marionette lines
   (Depressor anguli oris m.)
8. Chin line
   (Mentalis m.)

FIGURE 5 ● Wrinkles and folds of the face–oblique (contributing muscle). Copyright R. Small, MD.

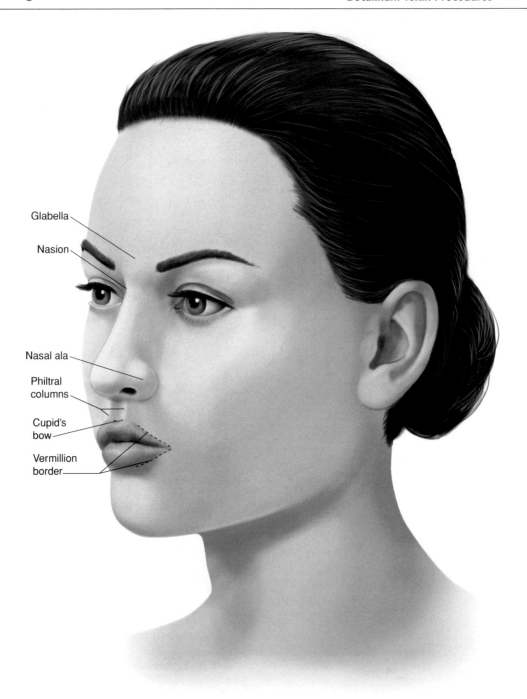

Glabella

Nasion

Nasal ala

Philtral
columns

Cupid's
bow

Vermillion
border

FIGURE 6 ● Surface anatomy of the face. Copyright R. Small, MD.

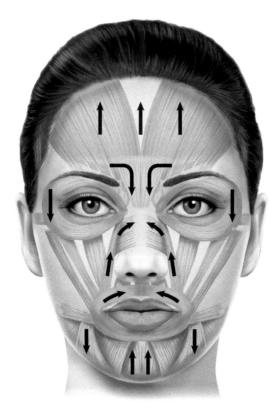

FIGURE 7 ● Functional anatomy of the face. Copyright R. Small, MD.

TABLE 1

EXPRESSION LINES	MUSCLES	ACTIONS
Frown lines	Corrugator supercilii	Eyebrows drawn medially
	Procerus and depressor supercilii	Medial eyebrow depressors
Horizontal forehead lines	Frontalis	Eyebrow levator
Crow's feet	Lateral orbicularis oculi	Lateral eyebrow depressor
Eyebrow lift	Superior lateral orbicularis oculi	Superior lateral eyebrow depressor
Bunny lines	Nasalis	Nasal sidewalls drawn medially
Radial lip lines	Orbicularis oris	Lip puckering
Marionette lines	Depressor anguli oris	Corner of mouth depressor
Nasolabial folds	Levator labii superioris alaeque nasi	Central lip levator
Chin line	Mentalis	Chin puckering and lower lip levator

Key:
Orange—depressor muscles   Purple—levator muscles   Gray—sphincteric muscles

Section 2

Introduction and Foundation Concepts

Administering botulinum toxin injections is an essential skill for physicians and qualified healthcare providers who wish to incorporate aesthetic medicine into their practice. According to statistics from the American Society of Plastic Surgeons, since its approval for cosmetic use by the U.S. Food and Drug Administration (FDA), botulinum toxin has become the most commonly performed minimally invasive cosmetic procedure, with over 3 million treatments performed annually. To successfully perform botulinum toxin procedures, an understanding of relevant anatomy and an appreciation for facial aesthetics, in addition to injection skill, are necessary to achieve desirable results.

Skin Aging

Wrinkling is a prominent feature of skin aging. Skin naturally thins and loses volume over time as dermal collagen, hyaluronic acid, and elastin gradually diminish. This process of dermal atrophy is accelerated and compounded by sun exposure and other extrinsic factors such as smoking. Hyperdynamic facial musculature also contributes to formation of visible lines and wrinkles. Initially, lines and wrinkles are seen only during active facial expression such as frowning, laughing, or smiling and are referred to as dynamic lines (Fig. 1A). Over time, dynamic lines become permanently etched into skin resulting in static lines (Fig. 2B), which are present at rest.

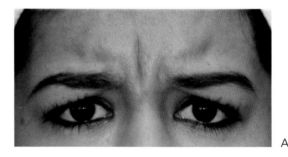

A

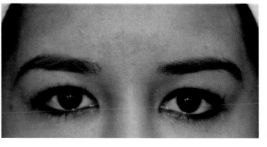

FIGURE 1 ● Younger patient demonstrating dynamic frown lines seen with glabellar complex muscle contraction **(A)** and lack of static lines at rest **(B)**. Copyright R. Small, MD.

B

9

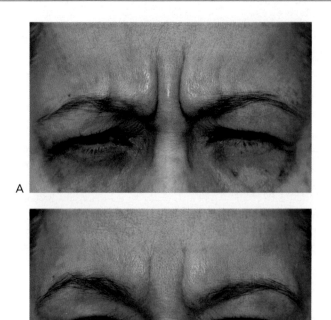

FIGURE 2 ● Older patient demonstrating dynamic frown lines seen with glabellar complex muscle contraction **(A)** and static lines at rest **(B)**. Copyright R. Small, MD.

Skin laxity, redistribution of facial fat, and biometric changes such as bone resorption, contribute to skin folds and facial contour changes. In addition, aged skin exhibits dyschromia such as mottled pigmentation, vascular ectasias such as telangiectasias and cherry angiomas, and undergoes benign and malignant degenerative changes.

Botulinum Toxin Indications (Year Approved)

- Botulinum toxin is FDA approved for the temporary treatment of moderate to severe dynamic glabellar frown lines in adults aged 18–65 years (2002).
- Botulinum toxin is FDA approved for the temporary treatment of primary axillary hyperhidrosis (2004).
- Other FDA approved indications include blepharospasm (1989), strabismus (1989), cranial nerve VII disorders (1989), cervical dystonia (2000), upper limb spasticity (2010), prophylaxsis for chronic migraine (2010).
- Other off-label cosmetic uses include reduction of wrinkles in the upper and lower face, neck, and chest; lifting of facial areas; and correction of facial asymmetries.

Mechanism of Action

Botulinum toxin is a neurotoxin protein derived from the *Clostridium botulinum* bacterium. When small quantities of botulinum toxin are injected into target muscles,

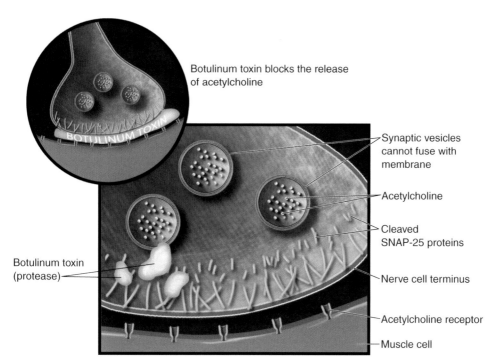

Botulinum toxin blocks the release of acetylcholine

Synaptic vesicles cannot fuse with membrane

Acetylcholine

Cleaved SNAP-25 proteins

Botulinum toxin (protease)

Nerve cell terminus

Acetylcholine receptor

Muscle cell

FIGURE 3 ● Botulinum toxin inhibits the release of acetylcholine at the neuromuscular junction. Copyright R. Small, MD.

localized chemical denervation occurs due to inhibition of acetylcholine release at the neuromuscular junction (Fig. 3). This temporarily reduces muscle contractions and smooths skin wrinkles in the treatment area.

Basic and Advanced Procedures

Basic. Areas of hyperdynamic muscles in the upper third of the face (frown lines, crow's feet and horizontal forehead lines) yield the most predictable results with the greatest efficacy, and fewest reported side-effects when treated with botulinum toxin. These areas are ideal for providers getting started with cosmetic botulinum toxin injections and are referred to as basic treatment areas (Table 1) in this book.

Advanced. Botulinum toxin treatments in the lower face are considered advanced procedures (Table 1). This is a highly functional region and, in addition to facial expression, lower face muscles serve essential functions of mastication and elocution. Treated muscles in the lower face must retain partial functionality which requires more practiced injection skill with precise placement of small doses of toxin. Botulinum toxin treatment of neck bands, hyperhidrosis and all facial areas other than the basic treatment areas, are considered advanced procedures in this book. These procedures have a greater risk of complications, and it is advisable for novice injectors to gain skill and confidence with basic procedures before proceeding to advanced botulinum toxin procedures.

Patient Selection

Patients with dynamic wrinkles that have minimal to no static component (Fig. 1) demonstrate the most dramatic improvements with botulinum toxin treatments. Results for

TABLE 1

Basic and Advanced Botulinum Toxin Treatment Areas

Expression Lines		
Common Name	**Medical Name**	**Muscles**
Basic		
Frown lines	Glabellar rhytids	Glabellar complex: corrugator supercilii, procerus, and depressor supercilii
Horizontal forehead lines	Frontalis rhytids	Frontalis
Crow's feet	Lateral canthal rhytids	Lateral orbital orbicularis oculi
Advanced		
Lower eyelid wrinkles	Infraocular rhytids	Inferior preseptal orbicularis oculi
Eyebrow lift	Reduction of ptotic eyebrows and dermatochalasis	Superior lateral orbital orbicularis oculi
Bunny lines	Nasal rhytids	Nasalis
Lip lines (smoker's or lipstick lines)	Perioral rhytids	Orbicularis oris
Marionette lines	Melomental folds	Depressor anguli oris
Downturned corners of the mouth	Depressed oral commissures	Depressor anguli oris
Nasolabial folds	Melolabial folds	Levator labii superioris alaeque nasi
Gummy smile	Gingival show	Levator labii superioris alaeque nasi
Chin line	Mental crease or labiomental crease	Mentalis
Chin puckering	Mentalis contraction	Mentalis
Neck bands	Platysmal bands	Platysma

patients with static wrinkles (Fig. 2) are slower and cumulative, and may require two to three consecutive treatments for significant improvements. Deep static lines may not fully respond to botulinum toxin treatment alone and may require combination treatment with dermal fillers or resurfacing procedures to achieve optimal results. Severe static wrinkles and laxity, commonly seen in patients aged 65 years or older, may require surgical intervention. Discussion regarding realistic expectations and results during the evaluation and consultation process is essential.

Treatment Goals

Botulinum toxin treatments are directed at specifically targeted muscles or regions of muscles to focally inhibit contraction and achieve intended effects such as smoothing the skin or elevating facial areas. An optimal result yields a pleasing aesthetic effect with minimal to no functional impairment in the treatment area and, lack of other undesired effects and complications.

The degree of muscle inhibition achieved with botulinum toxin in a given treatment area is determined by patient preference and the need to preserve functionality in the treated muscles. For example, some patients may desire complete inhibition of the glabellar complex muscles with botulinum toxin treatment of frown lines, whereas others may desire partial muscle inhibition with retention of some ability to frown. A greater degree of muscle inhibition is typically sought for treatments in the upper third of the face than in the lower face. In the lower face, partial muscle inhibition is the desired result as the treated muscles must still be able to perform essential functions, such as eating, drinking, and speaking. Treatment goals listed in the following chapters are based on common patient preferences and considerations of muscle functionality in the treatment areas.

Products

C. botulinum bacteria produce eight serotypes of botulinum toxin proteins (A, B, Cα, Cβ, D, E, F, and G). Botulinum toxin serotype A is the most potent and is used for cosmetic indications. The FDA currently approve two botulinum toxin serotype A products for the treatment of the glabellar complex muscles that form frown lines: onabotulinumtoxinA (OBTX) (Botox® manufactured by Allergan, Inc, Irvine, CA) and abobotulinumtoxinA (Dysport® manufactured by Medicis Pharmaceutical Corp, Scottsdale, AZ), both of which were formerly known as botulinum toxin type A. OBTX and abobotulinumtoxinA vary in formulation, diffusion capability, onset of action, efficacy, and complications and are not interchangeable. All references to OBTX in this book refer specifically to Botox.

Alternative Therapies

Botulinum toxin is the only treatment for dynamic wrinkles currently approved by the FDA. Other treatments for static wrinkles include chemical peels; microdermabrasion; topical products such as retinoids, nonablative lasers for soft-tissue coagulation and tightening such as infrared and radiofrequency; nonablative lasers for collagen remodeling such as 1320-nm, 1540-nm, and Q-switched lasers; ablative and fractional ablative lasers such as erbium and carbon dioxide lasers; and operative procedures such as dermabrasion and plastic surgery.

Contraindications

- Pregnancy or nursing
- Active infection in the treatment area (e.g., herpes simplex, pustular acne, cellulitis)
- Hypertrophic or keloidal scarring
- Bleeding abnormality (e.g., thrombocytopenia, anticoagulant use)
- Impaired healing (e.g., due to immunosuppression)
- Skin atrophy (e.g., chronic oral steroid use, genetic syndromes such as Ehlers-Danlos syndrome)
- Active dermatoses in the treatment area (e.g., psoriasis, eczema)
- Sensitivity or allergy to constituents of botulinum toxin (including botulinum toxin serotype A, human albumin, lactose, or sodium succinate)
- Milk allergy with abobotulinumtoxinA products
- Gross motor weakness in the treatment area (e.g., due to polio, Bell's palsy)
- Neuromuscular disorder including, but not limited to amyotrophic lateral sclerosis, myasthenia gravis, Lambert-Eaton syndrome, and myopathies

- Inability to actively contract muscles in the treatment area prior to treatment
- Periocular or ocular surgery within the previous 6 months (e.g., laser-assisted in situ keratomileusis, blepharoplasty)
- Medications that inhibit neuromuscular signaling and may potentiate botulinum toxin effects (e.g., aminoglycosides, penicillamine, quinine, calcium channel blockers)
- Uncontrolled systemic condition
- Occupation requiring uncompromised facial expression (e.g., actors, singers)
- Unrealistic expectations or body dysmorphic disorder

Advantages

- Technically straightforward with short treatment time
- Safe and effective, particularly in the upper third of the face
- High patient satisfaction

Disadvantage

- Short duration of action relative to other cosmetic procedures, although effects may be cumulative over time with recurring treatments

Equipment (Fig. 4)

- Botox reconstitution
  - Botox Cosmetic 100-unit vial
  - 5.0-mL syringe
  - 0.9% nonpreserved sterile saline 10-mL vial
  - 18-gauge, 0.5-inch needle
- Botox treatment
  - Reconstituted Botox Cosmetic (100 units/4 mL)
  - 1-mL Becton-Dickinson Luer-Lok™ tip syringe

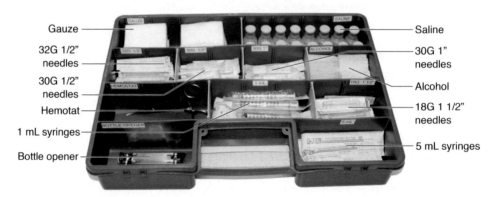

Gauze — 32G 1/2" needles — 30G 1/2" needles — Hemotat — 1 mL syringes — Bottle opener — Saline — 30G 1" needles — Alcohol — 18G 1 1/2" needles — 5 mL syringes

FIGURE 4 ● Equipment for botulinum toxin treatments. Copyright R. Small, MD.

- 30-gauge, 1-inch needle
- 30-gauge, 0.5-inch needle
- 32-gauge, 0.5-inch needle
- 3 × 3-inch nonwoven gauze
- Hand-held mirror (for consultation)
- Nonsterile gloves
- Alcohol pads
- Ice pack
- Bottle opener (for removing metal cap of the botulinum toxin vial for aspiration of fluid at the bottom of the vial)
- Hemostat (for loosening tight Luer-Lok connections)
- Soft, white eyeliner pencil or surgical pen (for marking injection points)

Reconstitution Method

Botox Cosmetic is supplied as a powder, typically in vials of 50 or 100 units. For reconstitution, non-preserved saline is recommended by the manufacturer and the author. Preserved saline is used for reconstitution by some providers because it may reduce discomfort with injection. There is no standardized volume for reconstitution. Botox efficacy is based on the number of units injected rather than the dilution. However, greater dilution volumes (of 10 mL or more) can increase diffusion and in turn the risk of complications.

The author's reconstitution method, using a 100-unit vial of Botox, is outlined as follows:

- Using an 18-gauge needle with a 5.0-mL syringe draw up 4.0 mL of 0.9% nonpreserved sterile saline.
- Insert the needle at a 45-degree angle into a 100-unit Botox vial and inject saline slowly, maintaining upward plunger pressure so that the diluent runs down the sides of the vial.
- Gently swirl the reconstituted Botox vial and record the date and time of reconstitution on the vial.
- Reconstitution of Botox powder using 4 mL of saline results in a concentration of 100 units of botulinum toxin per 4 mL (100 units/4 mL).

Reconstitution Concentrations and Dosing

Small volumes of reconstituted botulinum toxin solution are injected for cosmetic facial and neck treatments and a 1.0-mL syringe is used for injections. Providers must be aware of the exact dose associated with each 0.1-mL increment on the syringe for accurate dosing of botulinum toxin.

- With the earlier Botox reconstitution concentration of 100 units/4 mL:
  - 4.0 mL of reconstituted Botox has 100 units
  - 1.0 mL of reconstituted Botox has 25 units
  - 0.1 mL of reconstituted Botox has 2.5 units
- A table for conversion of botulinum toxin dose (in units) to injection volume (in mL) for Botox reconstituted at 100 units/4 mL is given in the appendix (Appendix 1, Table 1)

- Common reconstitution volumes used with a 100-unit vial of Botox and the resulting dose per 0.1 mL are shown below:

Saline Volume Added to 100-Unit Vial of Botox (mL)	Resulting Botulinum Toxin Dose Per 0.1 mL of Reconstituted Solution (Units)
1.0	10
2.0	5
2.5	4
4.0	2.5

Handling and Storage

Botox is shipped frozen, on dry ice. Before and after reconstitution it may be stored in the refrigerator at a temperature of 2–8°C (35.6–46.4°F) for up to 24–36 months based on the vial size. While the manufacturer recommends using Botox within 24 hours of reconstitution, the American Society for Plastic Surgery Botox Consensus Panel recommends using Botox within 6 weeks after reconstitution and notes no loss of potency during that time.

Anatomy

- Musculature of the face–anterior-posterior (Anatomy section, Fig. 1)
- Musculature of the face–oblique (Anatomy section, Fig. 2)
- Superficial and deep musculature of the face (Botulinum Toxin Anatomy section; Fig. 3)
- Wrinkles and folds of the face–anterior-posterior (Anatomy section, Fig. 4)
- Wrinkles and folds of the face–oblique (Anatomy section, Fig. 5)
- Surface anatomy of the face (Anatomy section, Fig. 6)
- Functional anatomy (Anatomy section, Fig. 7)

Understanding the facial anatomy in the treatment areas is necessary before performing botulinum toxin procedures (Anatomy section; Figs. 1–7). Most facial muscles have soft-tissue attachments to the skin through the superficial muscular aponeurotic system. When a muscle contracts, the overlying skin moves with it causing wrinkles (also called "rhytids") to form perpendicular to the direction of the muscle contraction. This allows for a diverse array of subtle facial expressions and functions.

Aesthetic Consultation

Review the patient's complete history, including medications, allergies, medical history including conditions contraindicating treatment, cosmetic history including minimally invasive aesthetic procedures and plastic surgeries as well as satisfaction with results and any side effects, and social history including occupations in which facial expression cannot be compromised.

Examine the areas of concern and, with the patient holding a mirror, have the patient prioritize the areas. Note any asymmetries, such as uneven eyebrow height, document in the chart and photograph. Discuss treatment options, number of recommended treatments, anticipated results, realistic expectations, and procedure cost. Review risks of complications associated with the procedure. Formulate a cosmetic treatment plan and record in the chart along with a consent form signed by the patient. It is advisable to use photographic documentation (referred to as photodocumentation) with aesthetic procedures and take dynamic and static photographs before botulinum toxin treatment and approximately 2 weeks posttreatment to demonstrate results.

When discussing botulinum toxin or other injection treatments, it can be helpful to use nonmedical or "patient friendly" terminology to reduce patient anxiety. Examples of terms used include the following:

Medical Terms	Patient-Friendly Terms
• Toxin	• Natural purified protein
• Paralyzes	• Relaxes
• Pain	• Discomfort

Preprocedure Checklist

- Perform an aesthetic consultation and obtain informed consent.
- Take pretreatment photographs with the patient actively contracting the muscles in the intended treatment area and with the muscles at rest.
- Document and discuss any notable asymmetries before treatment.
- Minimize bruising by discontinuation of aspirin, vitamin E, St. John's wort, and other similar-action dietary supplements including: ginkgo, evening primrose oil, garlic, feverfew, and ginseng for 2 weeks. Discontinue other nonsteroidal anti-inflammatory medications and alcohol consumption 2 days before treatment.
- For hyperhidrosis treatment, discontinue antiperspirant use 24 hours before treatment and see Hyperhidrosis chapter for other preprocedure steps.
- For the procedure, position the patient comfortably in a reclined position at about 65 degrees.
- Identify the *safety zone* for treatment, which is the recommended region within which injections are administered. Confining treatments to the safety zone area can maximize efficacy and minimize side effects.
- Locate the target muscles for botulinum toxin injection, which are located within the safety zone, by instructing the patient to contract the relevant muscles using particular facial expressions as outlined in each chapter.
- Identify the botulinum toxin injection points and OBTX starting doses from the overview figure, which accompanies each chapter.
- Instruct the patient to close their eyes during the procedure.
- Cleanse the treatment areas with alcohol prior to injection and allow alcohol to dry.

Anesthesia

Anesthesia is typically not required for botulinum toxin treatments. If necessary, ice or a topical anesthetic may be used before injections (e.g., benzocaine, lidocaine, tetracaine).

Pretreat the anesthetic injection sites with a topical anesthetic such as benzocaine 20% : lidocaine 6% : tetracaine 4% (BLT) for 15–20 minutes prior to treatment.

Commonly used topical anesthetic products include:
- L-M-X (lidocaine 4%–5%)*
- EMLA (lidocaine 2.5% : prilocaine 2.5%)**
- BLT (benzocaine 20% : lidocaine 6% : tetracaine 4%)***
  * Over-the-counter product   ** Prescription   ***Compounded by a pharmacy
  See Appendix 6, Supply Sources.

BLT is one of the most potent and fast acting topical anesthetics and is preferred for use by the author. It is applied in-office, with a maximum dose of 1/2 gm applied topically for 15 minutes. Effects are enhanced for certain topical anesthetics by occluding the product under plastic wrap once applied to the skin. Occlusion under plastic wrap is not necessary with BLT due to its potency.

Botulinum Toxin Dosing

- Each chapter has an overview figure of botulinum toxin injection points and recommended starting doses for a given treatment area using OBTX.
- Summary tables of starting doses for all treatment areas are provided in the appendix for OBTX (Appendix 1, Table 2a) and abobotulinumtoxinA (Appendix 1, Table 2b).

General Injection Techniques

- Insert the needle into the area of maximal muscle contraction, which is typically visible as a "hill" or "ridge" of muscle.
- The target for axillary hyperhidrosis is sweat glands located in the dermis. The targets for all other botulinum toxin treatments described in this book are muscles. In some facial areas, where the skin is thin and muscles are superficially located, subdermal injection adequately delivers botulinum toxin to the target muscle. In other areas deeper intramuscular injection is required.
- Depth of botulinum toxin injection is site specific and is either:
  - intradermal, visible as a wheal with dimpled skin (e.g., treatment of axillary hyperhidrosis);
  - subdermal, visible as a wheal without dimpled skin (e.g., treatment of crows feet); or
  - intramuscular, visible as a subtle wheal without dimpled skin or as mild edema in the injection area (e.g., treatment of frown lines).
- Botulinum toxin is typically injected as the needle is withdrawn and should flow very easily with minimal plunger pressure. If resistance is encountered, fully withdraw the needle and reinsert.
- Avoid intravascular injection. Intravascular injection is apparent when the surrounding skin blanches during injection. If this occurs, withdraw the needle partially from the blanched site, reposition, and inject.
- Avoid hitting the periosteum, particularly with frontalis muscle treatments, as this is painful and dulls the needle.
- After injecting, the site may be compressed to reduce discomfort and bleeding. When treating around the eye, compression is directed away from the eye.
- If bleeding occurs, achieve hemostasis before proceeding to subsequent injection points.
- Avoid vigorous massage of the area after treatment to minimize undesired dispersion of botulinum toxin to adjacent muscles.

- Changing needles after six or more injections maintains a sharp needle and minimizes discomfort.

Aftercare

On the day of treatment, instruct the patient to avoid lying down for 4 hours immediately after treatment, manipulating the treated area (e.g., a facial or massage), and activities that can cause facial flushing (e.g., application of heat to the face, alcohol consumption, exercising, and tanning) to reduce the likelihood of product migration and risk of side effects. If bruising or swelling occurs, a soft ice pack may be applied for 10–15 minutes to each bruise site, every 1–2 hours until it is improved.

Results and Follow-Up

- Treated muscles typically demonstrate partial reduction in function 2–3 days after botulinum toxin treatment, with maximal reduction 1–2 weeks after treatment. Effects are most noticeable for treatment of dynamic lines. Static lines are slower to respond, typically requiring two to three consecutive treatments and may need to be combined with other minimally invasive aesthetic procedures such as dermal fillers or resurfacing procedures to achieve optimal results.
- If desired reduction of muscle function is not achieved in the treatment area, a touch-up procedure may be performed 2 weeks after the initial treatment. The botulinum toxin touch-up dose varies according to the degree of movement remaining in the target muscles and the treatment area (see individual chapters for recommended touch-up doses). Reassess the treatment area 2 weeks after the touch-up procedure. Document and include photographs at each visit.
- Results of botulinum toxin treatments in the lower face are subtle, relative to the dramatic changes seen in the upper third of the face. Patients may be able to appreciate pre- and posttreatment improvements in dynamic lines of the lower face if they are schooled in how to make these assessments with animation. In addition to a pleasing aesthetic effect, a desirable result in the lower face also has minimal to no functional impairment of the mouth.
- Muscle function in the treatment area gradually returns 2–5 months after treatment, based on the dose of botulinum toxin used, treatment area and the patient's physiology. Subsequent treatments are recommended when muscles in the treated area begin to contract, prior to facial lines returning to their pretreatment appearance.

Learning the Techniques

- Marking the safety zone with a soft, white eyeliner pencil or surgical marker before treatment can help with locating the target muscles for treatment and marking the injection points can help with needle placement.
- It is advisable to start with conservative botulinum toxin doses; each chapter has recommended starting doses for a given treatment area.
- Consider performing initial treatments on staff and family to get feedback and to closely observe the effects of botulinum toxin.
- Touch-up procedures may be performed 2 weeks after initial treatment if necessary.
- Consider receiving a treatment to gain personal knowledge about botulinum toxin procedures.

Complications

Complications and side effects can be categorized into injection-related or botulinum toxin–related issues. Botulinum toxin–related complications listed below may be associated with treatment of the face and the neck. Complications associated with treatment of specific areas, as well as suggestions for management, are discussed in their respective chapters.

General Injection-Related Complications

- Pain
- Bruising
- Erythema
- Edema
- Tenderness
- Headache
- Infection
- Numbness or dysesthesia
- Anxiety
- Vasovagal episode and loss of consciousness

Pain with botulinum toxin injections is minimal as small-gauge needles are used for treatment. If necessary, injection pain can be reduced using ice, or topical anesthetics. Pretreatment anesthesia, especially with topical anesthetics, can prolong treatment times.

Bruising is commonly seen with botulinum toxin injections, particularly with treatment of crow's feet.. Bruises can range in size from pinpoint needle insertion marks to quarter-sized ecchymoses or, rarely, hematomas. The time for resolution of a bruise depends on the patients' physiology and the size of the bruise, where larger bruises can be visible for up to 1–2 weeks. Prevention of bruising is preferable and several suggestions for bruise prevention are listed in the Preprocedure Checklist above. Immediate application of ice and pressure to a bruise can minimize bruise formation. Bruises can be camouflaged after treatment with makeup.

Erythema and **edema** are seen with almost all injections and usually resolve within a few hours after treatment. Firm compression of injection sites, particularly on the forehead, can effectively reduce edema. Icing is not typically necessary for these issues.

Headaches can occur with upper face injections and usually resolve within a few days after treatment without medication. There are reports of idiosyncratic severe headaches lasting 2–4 weeks. Nonsteroidal anti-inflammatory medications are usually adequate for management of headaches.

Infection is rare with botulinum toxin injections but can occur with any procedure that breaches the skin. The most common etiologies are bacterial or reactivation of herpes simplex. Prolonged **pain, tenderness,** and **erythema,** of more than a few days' duration can signal infection and necessitates evaluation, with infection-specific treatment.

Numbness or **dysesthesia** in the treatment area is extremely rare and could result from nerve injury with injections.

Anxiety with injection procedures is common. Most patients have mild procedural anxiety, which can be reduced by ensuring that injection equipment is not visible during treatment and can be managed with breathing techniques. Rarely, patients with more severe anxiety may require preprocedural medications (e.g., tramadol 50 mg, 1 tablet 30 minutes prior to procedure). Vasovagal episodes associated with severe anxiety are possible, and it is advisable for offices to have emergency protocols when performing injection procedures.

Botulinum Toxin–Related Complications

- Localized burning or stinging pain during injection
- Blepharoptosis (droopy eyelid)
- Eyebrow ptosis (droopy eyebrow)
- Ectropion of the lower eyelid (eyelid margin eversion)
- Lagophthalmos (incomplete eyelid closure)
- Xerophthalmia (dry eyes)
- Epiphora (excess tearing)
- Diplopia (double vision)
- Impaired blink reflex
- Photophobia (light sensitivity)
- Globe trauma
- Infraorbital festooning (worsening of eye bags)
- Lip ptosis with resultant smile asymmetry
- Oral incompetence with resultant drooling and impaired speaking, eating, or drinking
- Cheek flaccidity
- Dysarthria (difficulty articulating)
- Dysphagia (difficulty swallowing), necessitating nasogastric tube placement in severe cases
- Hoarseness
- Neck weakness
- Facial asymmetry, alteration, or poor aesthetic result
- Inadequate reduction of wrinkles or lack of intended effect in the treatment area
- Worsening wrinkles in areas adjacent to the treatment area
- Weakening muscles adjacent to the treatment area
- Autoantibodies against botulinum toxin. Autoantibodies may be present or develop after injection, rendering treatments ineffective (1–2% of patients treated for cosmetic indications per Allergan)
- Extremely rare, immediate hypersensitivity reaction with signs of urticaria, edema, and a remote possibility of anaphylaxis
- Case reports of severe side effects due to distant spread from the site of injection have been reported with large doses of botulinum toxin, including: generalized muscle weakness, urinary incontinence, respiratory difficulties, and death due to respiratory compromise. These complications have been reported in patients hours to weeks after receiving large doses of botulinum toxin for noncosmetic indications (e.g., 300 units in the calf muscles). They have not been reported with cosmetic use of botulinum toxin at the labeled dose of 20 units (for glabellar lines) or 100 units (for primary axillary hyperhidrosis).

Some complications can be improved with botulinum toxin treatment of muscles that antagonize the affected muscles. However, for most complications, there are no corrective treatments and they spontaneously resolve as botulinum toxin effects diminish.

Utilizing precise injection technique into targeted muscles and minimizing diffusion of botulinum toxin with low reconstitution volumes, reduce involvement of adjacent muscles and decrease the likelihood of undesired effects and complications.

Botulinum Toxin Treatments in Multiple Facial Areas

Botulinum toxin treatments in the upper third of the face can be safely and easily combined with treatment in the lower face during a given visit.

Concomitant botulinum toxin treatment of multiple areas in the upper face may be performed; however, this can decrease expressivity. Some patients may, therefore, prefer to space out treatments in the upper face. For example, two areas may be treated together, such as the crow's feet and frown, and 1–2 months later, treatment of the forehead and an eyebrow lift may be performed.

The lower face is a highly functional region, responsible for speaking, eating, and drinking. Excessive weakening of the muscles in this region can result in significant complications from functional impairment and it is advisable to use caution when treating multiple areas in the lower face and the neck. A conservative approach is to rotate treatment areas every 3–4 months such that only one area is treated with botulinum toxin at any give time. For example, if botulinum toxin treatment of upper lip lines and mental crease are desired, then the orbicularis oris muscle may be treated initially, followed by treatment of the mentalis muscle 3 months later once the upper lip botulinum toxin effect has resolved.

New Products and Current Developments

IncobotulinumtoxinA (Xeomin® manufactured by Merz Pharmaceuticals, Greensboro, NC), and PurTox® (manufactured by Mentor Corporation, Santa Barbara, CA) are new injectable botulinum toxin products currently undergoing FDA approval for cosmetic use in the United States.

RT001 or ReVance (ReVance Therapeutics, Newark, CA) is a physician-applied topical botulinum toxin under investigation for cosmetic applications including treatment of the crow's feet and axillary hyperhidrosis.

Reimbursement and Financial Considerations

Cosmetic botulinum toxin treatments are not covered by insurance. Fees for botulinum toxin injections are usually based on the number of units used, or on the treatment site. Prices vary widely according to community pricing in different geographic regions and range from $10–$25 per unit or $250–$500 per site. The Current Procedural Terminology (CPT) designation for botulinum toxin procedures of the face is chemodenervation of muscles innervated by the facial nerve (CPT code 64612).

Combining Aesthetic Treatments

Facial aging is a multifaceted process involving not only the formation of facial lines and wrinkles but also contour changes, skin laxity, formation of dyschromic and vascular lesions, undesired hair growth, as well as benign and malignant degenerative changes. Achieving optimal rejuvenation results often requires a combination of treatments to address these different aspects of facial aging. Botulinum toxin can be easily combined with other minimally invasive aesthetic procedures such as dermal fillers to treat static lines and volume loss; lasers and intense pulsed light for hair reduction, skin resurfacing, and treatment of benign pigmented and vascular lesion; exfoliation procedures like microdermabrasion and chemical peels; and topical skin care products.

Minimally invasive aesthetic procedures like botulinum toxin offer patients a means to enhance their appearance in a subtle, natural way and maintain a healthy youthful appearance. From the provider's perspective, these procedures can be readily incorporated into practice to provide office-based aesthetic care.

Treatment Areas

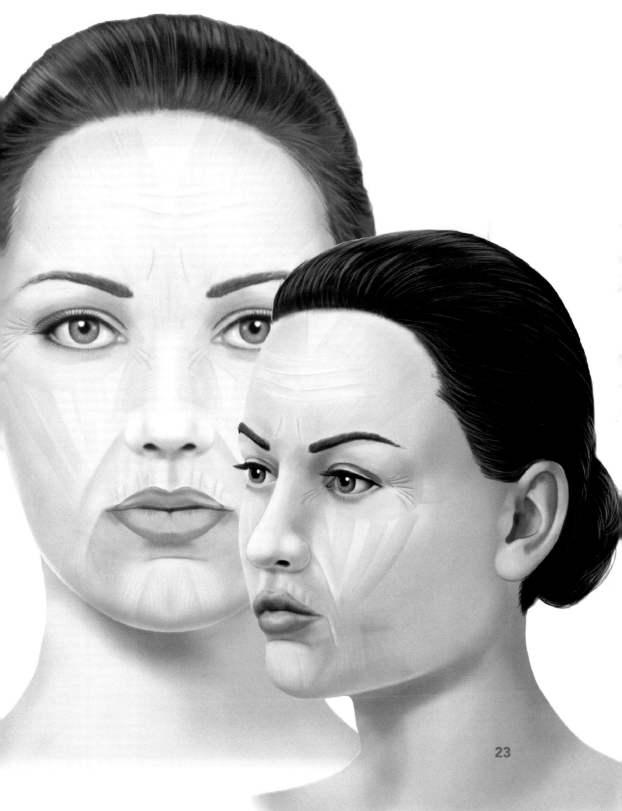

Chapter 1

Frown Lines

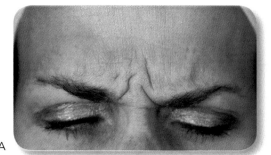 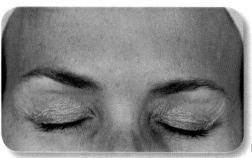

A

B

FIGURE 1 ● Frown lines before **(A)** and 1 month after **(B)** botulinum toxin treatment of the glabellar complex, with active frowning. Copyright R. Small, MD.

Dynamic frown lines result from contraction of glabellar complex muscles. These lines convey irritation, frustration, or anger and reduction of frown lines is one of the most common cosmetic complaints. Botulinum toxin treatment of the glabellar complex reduces frown lines by inhibiting contraction of these muscles and smoothing the overlying skin.

Indications

- Frown lines
- Medial eyebrow elevation

Anatomy

- **Wrinkles.** Frown lines, or glabellar rhytids, are vertical lines between the medial eyebrows (see Anatomy section, Figs. 4 and 5).
- **Muscles targeted**. Botulinum toxin frown line treatment targets the glabellar complex depressor muscles, which include the corrugator supercilii, procerus, and depressor supercilii (see Anatomy section, Figs. 1 and 2). The corrugator

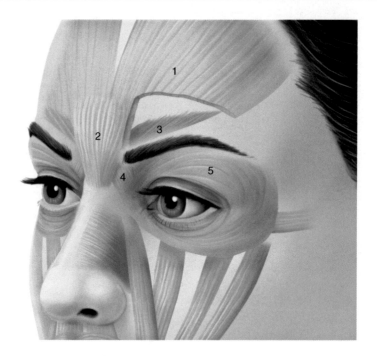

1. Frontalis m.   4. Depressor supercilii m.
2. Procerus m.   5. Orbicularis oculi m.
3. Corrugator supercilii m.

FIGURE 2 ● Glabellar complex detailed anatomy. Copyright R. Small,
MD.

and depressor supercilii muscles lie beneath the frontalis and procerus muscles
(Fig. 2).
• **Muscle functions.** Contraction of the glabellar complex muscles draws the eyebrows
  medially and inferiorly (see Anatomy section; Fig. 7 and Table 1).
• **Muscles avoided.** The portion of the frontalis muscle which is lateral to the corruga-
  tor muscles is avoided with treatment of the glabellar complex.

Patient Assessment

• **Dynamic** (with muscle contraction) and **static** (at rest) **frown lines** are assessed.
• **Concomitant frontalis and glabellar complex muscle contraction** with frowning
  (Fig. 3) are assessed. Patients who use both these muscle groups when frowning may
  require treatment of the frontalis in addition to treatment of the glabellar complex
  muscles to smooth frown lines.

Eliciting Contraction of Muscles to Be Treated

Instruct the patient to perform any of the following expressions:

• "Frown like you're mad"
• "Concentrate"

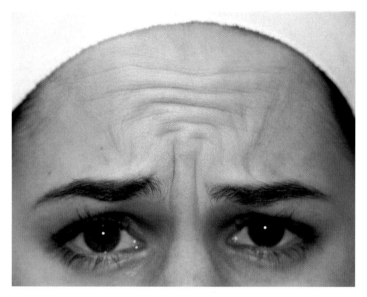

FIGURE 3 ● Frontalis and glabellar complex muscle contraction with frowning. Copyright R. Small, MD.

Treatment Goals

- Complete inhibition of glabellar complex muscles.

Reconstitution

- Reconstitute 100 units of Botox Cosmetic powder with 4 mL of nonpreserved saline (see Introduction and Foundation Concepts, Reconstitution Method section).
- Botulinum toxin products are not interchangeable and all references in this chapter to onabotulinumtoxinA (OBTX) refer specifically to Botox.

Starting Doses

- Women: 20 units of OBTX
- Men: 25 units of OBTX

Anesthesia

- Anesthesia is not necessary for most patients but an ice pack may be used if required.

Equipment for Treatment

- General botulinum toxin injection supplies (see Introduction and Foundation Concepts, Equipment)
- Reconstituted Botox Cosmetic
- 30-gauge, 1-inch needle

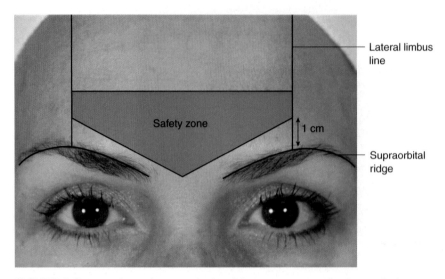

FIGURE 4 ● Frown line safety zone for botulinum toxin treatments. Copyright R. Small, MD.

Procedure Overview

- Place injections within the frown line safety zone (Fig. 4). The safety zone is at least 1 cm above the supraorbital ridge at the lateral limbus line, and extends inferiorly to a point approximately 1 cm below the glabellar prominence. It is bounded by vertical lines extending from the lateral limbi to the hairline.
- An overview of injection points and OBTX doses for treatment of frown lines is shown in Figure 5.
- Botulinum toxin is injected intramuscularly for treatment of frown lines.
- Injecting inferior to the safety zone, less than 1 cm above the supraorbital ridge at the lateral limbus line, increases the risk of blepharoptosis (droopy upper eyelid).

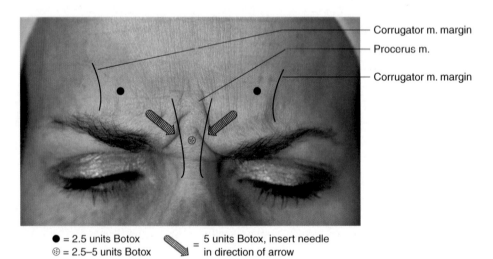

FIGURE 5 ● Overview of botulinum toxin injection points and doses for treatment of frown lines. Copyright R. Small, MD.

• Injecting lateral to the safety zone may involve the frontalis muscle, resulting in eyebrow ptosis (droopy eyebrow).

Technique

1. Position the patient at a 60-degree reclined position.
2. Identify the frown line safety zone (Fig. 4).
3. Locate the glabellar complex muscles and identify the lateral margins of the corrugators that lie within the safety zone by instructing the patient to contract the muscles, using one of the facial expressions above.
4. Identify the injection points (Fig. 5).
5. Ice for anesthesia (optional).
6. Prepare injection sites with alcohol and allow to dry.
7. The provider is positioned on the same side that is to be injected.
8. While the glabellar complex muscles are contracted, insert the needle 1–2 cm above the supraorbital ridge at the lateral margin of the corrugator muscle within the safety zone. Angle the needle towards the procerus muscle and insert to half the needle length (Fig. 6). Inject 2.5 units of OBTX with gentle, even plunger pressure as the needle is slowly withdrawn.

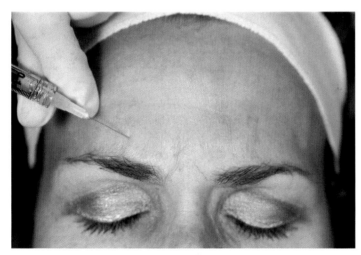

FIGURE 6 ● Lateral corrugator muscle botulinum toxin injection technique. Copyright R. Small, MD.

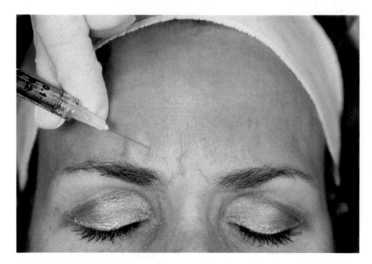

FIGURE 7 ● Medial corrugator muscle botulinum toxin injection technique. Copyright R. Small, MD.

9. The second injection point is placed deep in the body of the corrugator muscle, approximately 1 cm medial and inferior to the first injection point, closer to the eyebrow (Fig. 7). Angle the needle towards the procerus muscle and insert to the hub. Inject 5 units of OBTX as the needle is slowly withdrawn.
10. Repeat the above injections for the contralateral side of the face.
11. The third injection point is in the procerus muscle. Reposition to stand in front of the patient. While the glabellar complex muscles are contracted, approach inferiorly, direct the needle towards the glabella, insert to half the needle length, and inject 2.5–5 units of OBTX (Fig. 8).
12. Compress the injection sites firmly, directing pressure away from the eye.

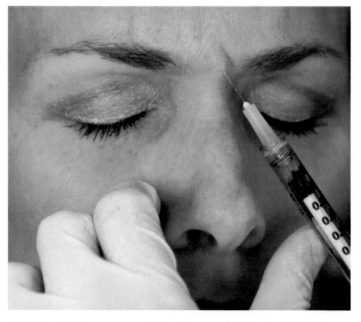

FIGURE 8 ● Procerus muscle botulinum toxin injection technique. Copyright R. Small, MD.

Results

- Reduction of dynamic frown lines is typically seen 3 days after botulinum toxin treatment, with maximal reduction at 1–2 weeks (Figs. 1A and 1B).

Duration of Effects and Treatment Intervals

- Muscle function in the treatment area gradually returns 3–4 months after botulinum toxin treatment.
- Subsequent frown line treatments with botulinum toxin may be performed when the glabellar complex muscles begin to contract, prior to lines returning to their pretreatment appearance.

Follow-Ups and Management

Patients are assessed 2 weeks after botulinum toxin treatment to evaluate for reduction of frown lines. If persistent frown lines are present, evaluate for the following common causes:

- **Glabellar muscle contraction.** Patients may have greater muscle mass than anticipated in the treatment area and additional botulinum toxin may be required to achieve desired results. Persistent muscle contraction can be corrected with a touch-up procedure using 5–10 units of OBTX, depending on the degree of glabellar muscle activity present.
- **Broad glabellar complex musculature.** If the lateral margins of the corrugators extend outside the safety zone lines these portions of the corrugators will not receive treatment. These untreated portions of the corrugators retain function and may cause medial frown lines. Treating these active lateral portions of the corrugators is not advisable because of the risks of blepharoptosis and eyebrow ptosis.
- **Frontalis muscle contraction with frowning.** In some patients, frontalis muscle contraction contributes to frown line formation and botulinum toxin treatment of the frontalis may be required to achieve optimal frown line reduction.
- **Static lines.** Patients with superficial static lines that do not have an underlying depression may require several consecutive botulinum toxin treatments for results to be seen. Patients with deep static lines that have an underlying depression often benefit from combining botulinum toxin with dermal fillers (see Combining Aesthetic Treatments below).

Complications and Management

- General injection-related complications (see Introduction and Foundation Concepts, Complications)
- Blepharoptosis (droopy eyelid)
- Eyebrow ptosis (droopy eyebrow)

Blepharoptosis is a temporary complication that can occur with botulinum toxin treatment of the glabellar complex muscles, particularly if toxin is injected too close to the supraorbital ridge at the lateral limbus line. Figure 9 shows a patient 3 weeks after botulinum toxin treatment (not by the author) to glabellar complex muscles with a profound right-sided blepharoptosis and mild right eyebrow ptosis. Blepharoptosis is typically seen as a 2–3-mm lowering of the affected eyelid, which is most marked at the end of the day with muscle fatigue. It is infrequent (1–5%), almost always unilateral, and usually resolves spontaneously within 6 weeks.

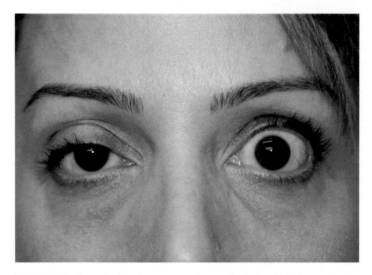

FIGURE 9 ● Right blepharoptosis. Copyright R. Small, MD.

Blepharoptosis results from migration of botulinum toxin through the orbital septum fascia to the levator palpebrae superioris muscle in the upper eyelid. Some of the levator palpebrae superioris muscle fibers pass up through the orbital septum to attach on the supraorbital ridge at the lateral limbus, and botulinum toxin can migrate into the levator palpebrae superioris at this point.

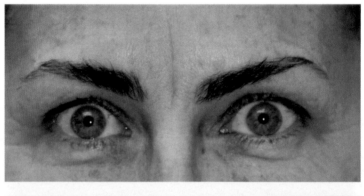

A

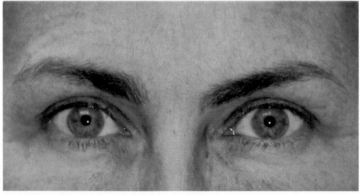

B

FIGURE 10 ● Deep static frown line before **(A)** and 1 month after **(B)** combination treatment with botulinum toxin in the glabellar complex and dermal filler in the frown line. Copyright R. Small, MD.

Blepharoptosis can be treated using over-the-counter alpha-adrenergic eye drops, such as naphazoline/pheniramine (e.g., Naphcon-A, one drop four times per day in the affected eye) or with prescription apraclonidine 0.5% solution (e.g., Iopidine, one to two drops three times per day). Both of these medications cause contraction of Mueller's muscle, an adrenergic levator muscle of the upper eyelid, resulting in elevation of the upper eyelid. Iopidine is reserved for refractory cases and should be used with caution as it can exacerbate or unmask underlying glaucoma.

- **Eyebrow ptosis** can result from relaxation of the lateral frontalis muscle, if botulinum toxin is injected lateral to the lateral limbus lines.

Combining Aesthetic Treatments and Maximizing Results

- **Deep static frown lines** associated with an underlying depression usually respond to a combination of botulinum toxin and dermal filler treatments. Figure 10 shows a deep static frown line before (Fig. 10A) and 1 month after (Fig. 10B) combination treatment with botulinum toxin in the glabellar complex and dermal filler treatment of the volume deficit.

Pricing

Charges for botulinum toxin treatment of frown lines range from $200–$500 per treatment or $10–$25 per unit of OBTX.

Chapter 2

Horizontal Forehead Lines

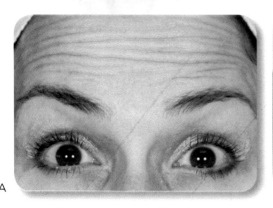
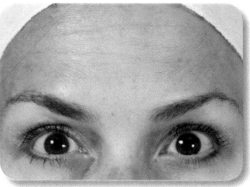

A   B

FIGURE 1 ● Horizontal forehead lines before **(A)** and 1 month after **(B)** botulinum toxin treatment of the frontalis muscle, with eyebrow elevation. Copyright R. Small, MD.

Dynamic horizontal forehead lines result from contraction of the frontalis muscle. Botulinum toxin treatment of the frontalis reduces forehead lines by inhibiting muscle contraction and smoothing the overlying skin. Frontalis muscle contraction also affects eyebrow shape and height, and certain botulinum toxin injection techniques in this area can result in lateral eyebrow elevation.

Indications

- Horizontal forehead lines
- Lateral eyebrow elevation

Anatomy

- **Wrinkles.** Horizontal forehead lines, or frontalis rhytids, course across the forehead (see Anatomy section, Figs. 4 and 5).
- **Eyebrow position and shape.** In women, high arched eyebrows are usually desired. In men, a flat eyebrow shape is usually preferable (see Eyebrow Lift chapter, Figs. 2A and 2B).
- **Muscles targeted.** Botulinum toxin horizontal forehead line treatment targets the broad frontalis muscle, which spans the forehead attaching laterally at the temporal fusion lines (see Anatomy section, Figs. 1 and 2).

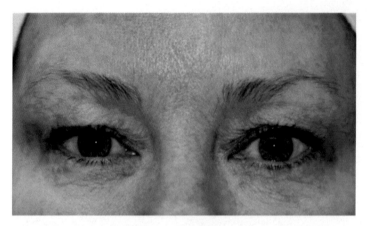

FIGURE 2 ● Dermatochalasis of the upper eyelid is a contraindication to horizontal forehead line treatment. Copyright R. Small, MD.

- **Muscle functions.** Frontalis muscle fibers are oriented vertically and contraction of this levator muscle raises the eyebrows. The inferior 2-cm portion has the most significant effect on eyebrow height and shape (see Anatomy section, Fig. 7 and Table 1).

Patient Assessment

- **Dynamic** (with muscle contraction) and **static** (at rest) **horizontal forehead lines** are assessed.
- **Dynamic and static eyebrow shape** is assessed.
- **Eyebrow ptosis** (low-set, droopy eyebrows) and **upper eyelid dermatochalasis** (skin laxity or redundancy) are assessed with the frontalis muscle at rest. Figure 2 shows a patient with significant upper eyelid dermatochalasis. Patients with these conditions often have horizontal forehead lines as frontalis muscle contraction is compensatory to elevate low set eyebrows and reduce upper eyelid skin laxity. While treatment with botulinum toxin will improve forehead lines, it can worsen these other conditions and, when getting started with botulinum toxin injections, it is advisable to avoid treatment in patients with dermatochalasis and eyebrow ptosis. As experience is gained with injection placement and dosing in this area, providers may choose to treat patients with these more challenging presentations.

Eliciting Contraction of Muscles to Be Treated

Instruct the patient to perform any of the following expressions:

- "Raise your eyebrows up like you're surprised"
- "Lift up your forehead"

Treatment Goals

- Complete inhibition of the medial frontalis muscle to reduce horizontal forehead lines with partial inhibition of the lateral frontalis muscle in order to maintain a desirable eyebrow shape.

Reconstitution

- Reconstitute 100 units of Botox Cosmetic powder with 4 mL of nonpreserved saline (see Introduction and Foundation Concepts section, Reconstitution Method)
- Botulinum toxin products are not interchangeable and all references in this chapter to onabotulinumtoxinA (OBTX) refer specifically to Botox.

Starting Doses

- Women: 15–22.5 units of OBTX
- Men: 20–25 units of OBTX

Anesthesia

- Anesthesia is not necessary for most patients but an ice pack may be used if required.

Equipment for Treatment

- General botulinum toxin injection supplies (see Introduction and Foundation Concepts section, Equipment)
- Reconstituted Botox Cosmetic
- 30-gauge, 0.5-inch needle

Procedure Overview

- Place injections within the horizontal forehead line safety zone (Fig. 3). The safety zone is bounded by vertical lines at the lateral limbi and includes the area 2 cm above the supraorbital ridge to the hairline, as well as a small area lateral to the vertical lines approximately 2 cm inferior to the hairline. Confining treatment to the safety zone minimizes the risk of eyebrow ptosis and preserves eyebrow shape and height.

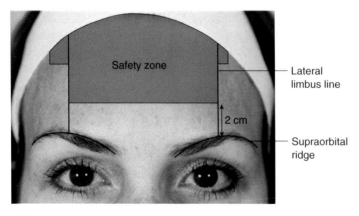

FIGURE 3 ● Horizontal forehead line safety zone for botulinum toxin treatments. Copyright R. Small, MD.

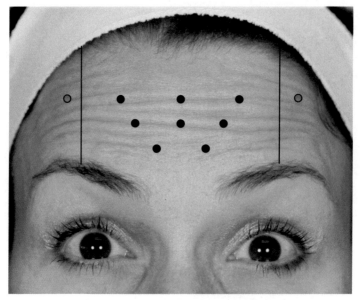

● = 1.25–2.5 units Botox   ● = 2.5 units Botox

FIGURE 4 ● Overview of botulinum toxin injection points and doses for treatment of horizontal forehead lines. Copyright R. Small, MD.

- An overview of injection points and OBTX doses for treatment of horizontal forehead lines is shown in Figure 4.
- Botulinum toxin is injected intramuscularly for treatment of horizontal forehead lines.
- Botulinum toxin placement and dosing lateral to the limbus lines can be tricky. Injecting inferior to the safety zone in this region or using high doses increases the risk of lateral eyebrow ptosis. However, botulinum toxin placed too superiorly near the hairline or use of very small doses may result in a peaked eyebrow shape. In general, it is better to have a result with peaked eyebrows (which can be corrected) than eyebrow ptosis.
- The "v-shaped" injection pattern shown in Figure 4 minimizes botulinum toxin injection in the lateral portion of the frontalis muscle and helps to preserve the eyebrow arch by elevating the lateral eyebrow, which is desirable for women. A flatter eyebrow shape can be achieved by injecting botulinum toxin a bit more inferiorly in the lateral frontalis.
- Injecting inferior to the safety zone between the limbus lines increases the risk of medial eyebrow ptosis.
- Avoid injecting too deeply and thus hitting the periosteum, which is painful and dulls the needle.

Technique

1. Position the patient at a 60-degree reclined position.
2. Identify the horizontal forehead safety zone (Fig. 3).

3. Locate the frontalis muscle and identify the ridges of the frontalis muscle by instructing the patient to contract the muscles, using one of the facial expressions above.
4. Identify the injection points (Fig. 4).
5. Ice for anesthesia (optional).
6. Prepare injection sites with alcohol and allow to dry.
7. The provider is positioned in front of the patient.
8. While the frontalis muscle is contracted, insert the needle into the frontalis muscle within the safety zone lines. The needle is angled at 30-degrees to the forehead and the tip is inserted into the muscle ridge. Inject 2.5 units of OBTX with gentle, even plunger pressure (Fig. 5).

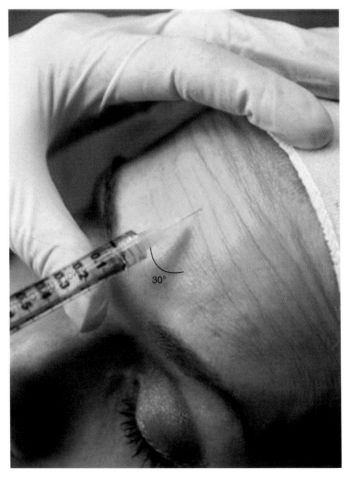

FIGURE 5 ● Medial frontalis muscle botulinum toxin injection technique. Copyright R. Small, MD.

9. Continue laterally along each ridge of frontalis muscle within the safety zone lines, injecting 2.5 units of OBTX approximately 1 cm apart. Perform injections evenly across the forehead to achieve symmetry (Fig. 6).
10. The final injection is placed just lateral to the safety zone line approximately 2 cm below the hairline, at the maximal point of eyebrow elevation. Inject 1.25–2.5 units of OBTX and repeat for the contralateral side.
11. Compress the injection sites firmly, directing pressure lateral to the safety zone line away from the eye.

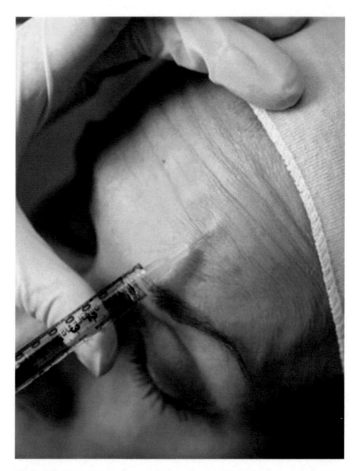

FIGURE 6 ● Frontalis muscle botulinum toxin injection technique.
Copyright R. Small, MD.

Results

- **Reduction of dynamic horizontal forehead lines** and **lateral eyebrow elevation** are typically seen 3 days after botulinum toxin treatment with maximal improvement at 1–2 weeks (Figs. 1A and 1B).

Duration of Effects and Treatment Intervals

- Muscle function in the treatment area gradually returns 3–4 months after treatment.
- Subsequent horizontal forehead line treatments with botulinum toxin may be performed when the frontalis muscle begins to contract before the lines return to their pretreatment appearance.

Follow-Ups and Management

Patients are assessed 2 weeks after botulinum toxin treatment to evaluate for reduction of forehead lines and eyebrow symmetry and eyebrow shape at rest and with active eyebrow elevation.

- **Peaked Eyebrow Shape or "Quizzical Brow".** Peaked eyebrows are most noticeable with animation and are due to excessive contraction of the lateral frontalis muscle. This can occur in patients with strong lateral frontalis muscles, if lateral frontalis muscle injections have been omitted, or if small botulinum toxin doses have been injected too superiorly in the lateral frontalis. Peaked eyebrows can be corrected with 1.25–2.5 units of OBTX placed just inferior to the lateral safety zone, in line with the most peaked portion of the eyebrow. Figure 7 shows a patient actively contracting the frontalis muscle demonstrating mildly peaked eyebrows bilaterally 2 weeks after treatment with 22.5 units of OBTX in the frontalis muscle and injection points for correction. Figure 1B shows the same patient 2 weeks after receiving 1.25 units of OBTX above each peaked eyebrow (4 weeks after the initial treatment) and represents the final result.

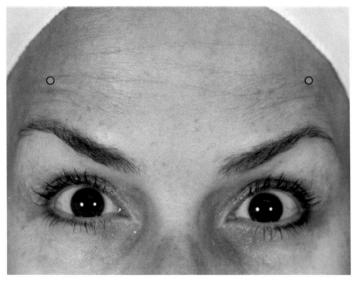

● = 1.25–2.5 units Botox

FIGURE 7 ● Peaked eyebrows and correction with botulinum toxin.
Copyright R. Small, MD.

Complications and Management

- General injection-related complications (see Introduction and Foundation Concepts section, Complications)
- Eyebrow ptosis (droopy eyebrow)
- Eyebrow asymmetry
- Blepharoptosis (droopy upper eyelid)

Eyebrow ptosis is one of the most significant complications from botulinum toxin treatment of the frontalis muscle. Excessive botulinum toxin dosing in the frontalis muscle or placement inferior to the safety zone can result in eyebrow ptosis. Patients often present with a complaint of heaviness of the upper eyelid on the affected side. Eyebrow ptosis may be unilateral or bilateral and is typically seen as a lowering and flattening of the affected eyebrow, while the palpebral fissures are unaffected and symmetric (unlike with blepharoptosis, where the palpebral fissure on the affected side is reduced). The medial, lateral, or entire eyebrow may be affected, depending on the region of frontalis muscle that is involved. Figure 8 shows a patient before (Fig. 8A)

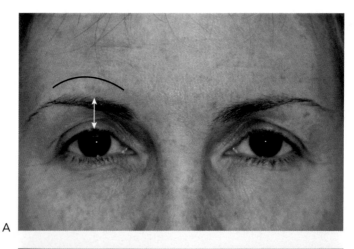

A

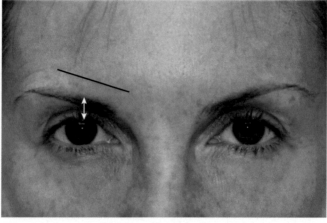

B

FIGURE 8 ● Eyebrow position before **(A)** and 2 weeks after **(B)** botulinum toxin treatment of the frontalis muscle demonstrating eyebrow ptosis. Copyright R. Small, MD.

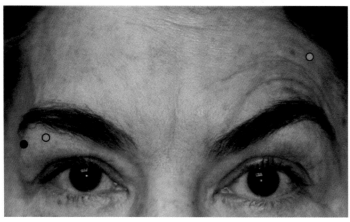

O = 1.25 units Botox   ● = 2.5 units Botox   ◐ = 1.25–2.5 units Botox

FIGURE 9 ● Eyebrow asymmetry and correction with botulinum toxin.
Copyright R. Small, MD.

and 2 weeks after (Fig. 8B) botulinum toxin treatment with 20 units of OBTX in the frontalis muscle demonstrating medial eyebrow ptosis. Eyebrow ptosis resolves spontaneously as botulinum toxin effects wear off. Medial eyebrow ptosis may be improved by treating the glabellar complex with botulinum toxin if this area is untreated (see Frown Lines chapter). Lateral eyebrow ptosis may be improved by treating the superior lateral orbicularis oculi with botulinum toxin and lifting the lateral eyebrow (see Eyebrow Lift chapter).

Eyebrow asymmetry may result from eyebrow ptosis and/or a peaked eyebrow. Figure 9 shows eyebrow asymmetry 2 weeks after botulinum toxin treatment with 22.5 units of OBTX in the frontalis muscle. The patient has a lower, flattened right eyebrow and a peaked left eyebrow. This asymmetry may be corrected by treating the superior lateral orbicularis oculi on the right side with botulinum toxin to lift the lateral eyebrow (see Eyebrow lift chapter), and treating the lateral frontalis on the left side to reduce the peaked eyebrow.

Blepharoptosis is uncommon with frontalis muscle treatments. It can result from inferior placement of botulinum toxin at the lateral limbus line with diffusion into the levator muscles of the upper eyelid. See Frown Lines chapter, Complications, for additional information on blepharoptosis and management strategies.

Combining Aesthetic Treatments and Maximizing Results

- **Eyebrow position and height** can be optimized by balancing depressor and levator muscle effects on the eyebrows with botulinum toxin treatments. Botulinum toxin treatment of the eyebrow depressor muscles, such as the glabellar complex (see Frown lines chapter) and superior lateral orbicularis oculi muscles (see Eyebrow lift chapter), complement botulinum toxin treatment of the frontalis levator muscle and reduce the risk of eyebrow ptosis.

- **Deep static horizontal forehead line** results can be enhanced by combining botulinum toxin treatments with resurfacing procedures such as fractional ablative lasers or chemical peels.

Pricing

Charges for botulinum toxin treatment of horizontal forehead lines range from $200–$500 per treatment or $10–$25 per unit of OBTX.

Chapter 3

Crow's Feet

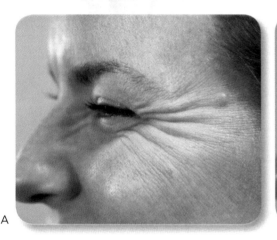
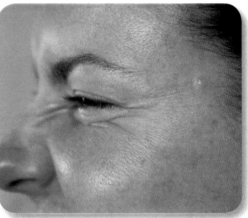

A   B

FIGURE 1 ● Crow's feet before **(A)** and 1 month after **(B)** lateral orbicularis oculi muscle botulinum toxin treatment, with active muscle contraction. Copyright R. Small, MD.

Dynamic crow's feet result from contraction of the orbicularis oculi muscle. Treatment of the lateral orbicularis oculi muscle with botulinum toxin inhibits contraction, reducing crow's feet and elevating the lateral eyebrow.

Indications

- Crow's feet
- Lateral eyebrow lift

Anatomy

- **Wrinkles.** Crow's feet, or lateral canthal rhytids, radiate laterally from the eye (see Anatomy section, Figs. 4 and 5).
- **Muscles targeted.** Botulinum toxin crow's feet treatment targets the lateral portion of the orbital orbicularis oculi muscle. The orbicularis oculi muscle is a superficial, thin, sphincteric muscle, which encircles the eye (see Anatomy section, Figs. 1 and 2). It has a palpebral portion covering the eye and an orbital portion around the eye (see Lower Eyelid Wrinkles chapter, Fig. 3).

- **Muscle functions.** Different regions of the orbicularis oculi muscle have different functions (see Anatomy section, Fig. 7 and Table 1). The lateral orbital portion of the orbicularis oculi muscle functions as a lateral eyebrow depressor (see Eyebrow Lift chapter) and contributes to formation of crow's feet. The palpebral portion of the orbicularis oculi muscle functions to close the eyelid both voluntarily and as part of the blink reflex. Lacrimal function, with lacrimal flow from the superior lateral gland to the medial lacrimal sac, is dependent on overall orbicularis oculi muscle strength.
- **Muscles avoided.** The lip levator muscles lie deep to the orbicularis oculi muscle and are avoided with treatment of crow's feet. The upper lip levators include the zygomaticus major and minor which are located near the lateral portion of the orbicularis oculi muscle at the superior margin of the zygomatic arch (see Anatomy section; and the levator labii superioris, levator labii superioris alaeque nasi, and levator anguli oris muscles which are located medially (see Anatomy section, Figs. 1, 2, and 3).

Patient Assessment

- **Blepharoplasty** and other facial surgery history is reviewed. Surgically altered anatomy may increase the risk of complications such as lip ptosis from lip levator muscle involvement. Ophthalmologic history, including keratorefractive (LASIK) surgery, is obtained as this may increase the risk of dry eyes.
- **Dynamic** (with muscle contraction) and **static** (at rest) crow's feet are assessed.

Eliciting Contraction of Muscles to Be Treated

Instruct the patient to perform any of the following expressions:

- "Make a cheesy grin" or "make a big smile"
- "Squint like the sun is in your eyes"
- "Wink"

Treatment Goals

- Complete inhibition of the lateral orbicularis oculi muscle.

Reconstitution

- Reconstitute 100 units of Botox Cosmetic powder with 4 mL of nonpreserved saline (see Introduction and Foundation Concepts section, Reconstitution Method).
- Botulinum toxin products are not interchangeable and all references in this chapter to onabotulinumtoxinA (OBTX) refer specifically to Botox.

Starting Doses

- Women: total (bilateral) dose is 15–20 units of OBTX
- Men: total (bilateral) dose is 20–25 units of OBTX

Anesthesia

- Anesthesia with ice is not recommended as it vasoconstricts and can obscure blood vessels.

Equipment for Treatment

- General botulinum toxin injection supplies (see Introduction and Foundation Concepts section, Equipment)
- Reconstituted Botox Cosmetic
- 30- or 32-gauge, 0.5-inch needle

Procedure Overview

- Place injections within the crow's feet safety zone (Figs. 2A and 2B). The safety zone is 1 cm outside the orbital rim, above the level of the superior margin of the zygoma and extends under the eyebrow to the lateral limbus line. Botulinum toxin is concentrated within the central crow's feet safety zone, but injections may also be placed in the extended safety zone according to patients' anatomy.

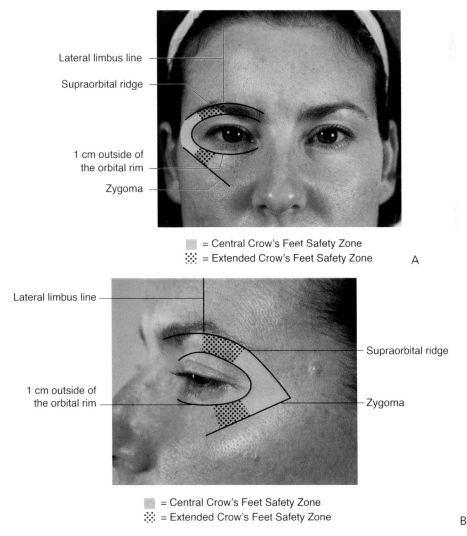

Lateral limbus line

Supraorbital ridge

1 cm outside of the orbital rim

Zygoma

■ = Central Crow's Feet Safety Zone
⋮⋮ = Extended Crow's Feet Safety Zone   A

Lateral limbus line

Supraorbital ridge

1 cm outside of the orbital rim

Zygoma

■ = Central Crow's Feet Safety Zone
⋮⋮ = Extended Crow's Feet Safety Zone   B

FIGURE 2 ● Crow's feet safety zone for botulinum toxin treatments: front **(A)** and lateral **(B)** views. Copyright R. Small, MD.

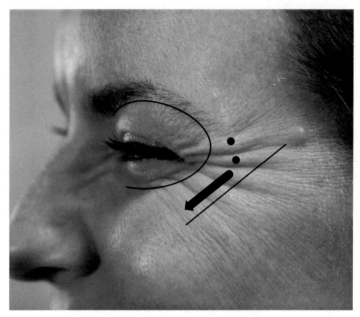

= 2.5 units Botox, insert needle in direction of arrow

FIGURE 3 ● Overview of botulinum toxin injection points and doses
for treatment of crow's feet. Copyright R. Small, MD.

- An overview of injection points and OBTX doses for treatment of crow's feet is shown in Figure 3. Injection points are located at the "ridges" of contracted muscle.
- Patterns of crow's feet vary; some extend superiorly toward the eyebrow and others extend inferiorly toward the cheek. Optimal treatment of the crow's feet is achieved by adapting the injection technique below to the patient's specific crow's feet pattern.
- Botulinum toxin is injected subdermally for treatment of crow's feet. It is important to place injections superficially in this region as the orbicularis oculi muscle overlies other muscles, which, if affected by botulinum toxin, can result in lip ptosis and other more serious complications. Subdermal injection can be achieved using the following technique: instruct the patient to contract the muscle in the treatment area by smiling and insert the needle just below the skin. Once the needle tip is inserted, instruct the patient to relax the muscle by slowly releasing their smile, and inject botulinum toxin to raise a visible wheal. The wheal is more visible at rest.
- The lateral canthal region has many veins and bruising is common. Veins are best seen and avoided using oblique lighting. If numerous vessels are visible in the treatment area, ecchymosis may be reduced by injecting a series of continuous wheals, where each injection is placed at the border of the previous wheal.
- Injecting superior to the crow's feet safety zone near the lateral limbus line at the orbital rim, can be associated with botulinum toxin migration into the levator muscles of the upper eyelid, resulting in blepharoptosis.

- Injecting medial to the crow's feet safety zone near the orbital rim at the lateral canthus, can be associated with deep migration of botulinum toxin into extraocular muscles, resulting in diplopia.
- Injecting deeply and inferior lateral to the crow's feet safety zone below the superior margin of the zygoma, may involve the lip levator muscles and increase the risk of cheek and lip ptosis, smile asymmetry, and possibly oral incompetence.
- Injecting deeply and inferior medial to the crow's feet safety zone may involve other lip levator muscles and increase the risk of cheek and lip ptosis, smile asymmetry, and profound oral incompetence.

Technique

1. Position the patient at a 60-degree reclined position.
2. Identify the crow's feet safety zone and palpate the orbital rim (Fig. 2).
3. Locate the orbicularis oculi muscle by instructing the patient to contract the muscles using one of the facial expressions above.
4. Identify the injection points (Fig. 3).
5. Prepare injection sites with alcohol and allow to dry.
6. The provider is positioned on the side that is to be injected.
7. While the lateral orbicularis oculi muscle is contracted, insert the needle 1 cm outside the orbital rim, near the lateral canthal line into the first injection point located at the muscle "ridge". The needle is inserted subdermally using the technique described earlier in the Procedure Overview. Inject 2.5 units of OBTX with gentle plunger pressure (Fig. 4).

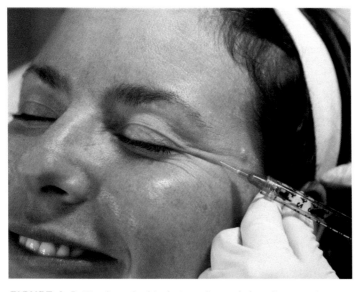

FIGURE 4 ● First lateral orbicularis oculi muscle botulinum toxin injection. Copyright R. Small, MD.

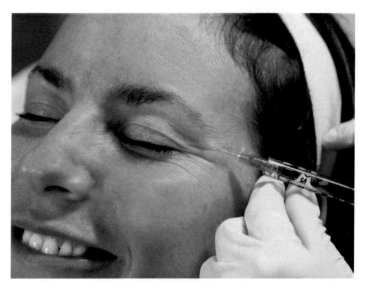

FIGURE 5 ● Second lateral orbicularis oculi muscle botulinum toxin injection. Copyright R. Small, MD.

8. The second injection point is approximately 0.5 cm superior to the first injection point. Inject 2.5 units of OBTX (Fig. 5).
9. The third injection point is approximately 0.5 cm inferior to the first injection point. The needle is angled inferiorly and threaded superficially to the hub. Inject 2.5 units of OBTX as the needle is withdrawn (see Fig. 6).
10. Repeat injections for the contralateral orbicularis oculi muscle.
11. Compress the injection sites firmly, directing pressure away from the eye.

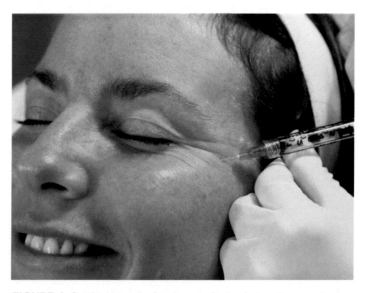

FIGURE 6 ● Third lateral orbicularis oculi muscle botulinum toxin injection. Copyright R. Small, MD.

Results

- **Reduction of dynamic crow's feet** and **lateral eyebrow elevation** is typically seen 3 days after botulinum toxin treatment, with maximal improvements at 1–2 weeks (see Figs. 1A and 1B).

Duration of Effects and Treatment Intervals

- Muscle function in the treatment area gradually returns 2.5–3 months after botulinum toxin treatment.
- Subsequent crow's feet treatments with botulinum toxin may be performed when the orbicularis oculi muscle begins to contract, before the lines return to their pretreatment appearance.

Follow-Ups and Management

Patients are assessed 2 weeks after botulinum toxin treatment to evaluate for reduction of crow's feet.

- **Persistent crow's feet.** If persistent crow's feet are present, evaluate for the following common causes:

  - **Orbicularis oculi muscle contraction.** Patients may have greater muscle mass than anticipated in the treatment area and additional botulinum toxin may be required to achieve desired results. Persistent muscle contraction can be corrected with a touch-up procedure using 2.5–10 units of OBTX, depending on the degree of orbicularis oculi muscle activity present. Reassess the treatment area 2 weeks after the touch-up procedure.
  - **Cheek muscle contraction.** Some patients will retain a few wrinkles inferior to the crow's feet treatment area, which are most noticeable with smiling (see Fig. 1B). These wrinkles are due to appropriately retained function of the zygomatic muscles and require no additional treatment.
  - **Static lines.** If static crow's feet are present, patients may require several consecutive botulinum toxin treatments for results to be seen. Combining botulinum toxin with other minimally invasive aesthetic procedures can offer enhanced results for treatment of static crow's feet (see Combining Aesthetic Treatments below).

- **Adjacent muscle involvement.** Some patients may complain of accentuated wrinkles in adjacent untreated areas, such as bunny lines on the nose, wrinkles under eyebrows or under the lower eyelids.

  - **Bunny lines** are readily treated with botulinum toxin in the nasalis muscle (see Bunny lines chapter).
  - **Lines under the eyebrow.** The infrabrow region contains the superior lateral orbicularis oculi muscle, which is not treated as part of botulinum toxin treatment for crow's feet. In some patients, wrinkles under the eyebrow may form due to compensatory contraction of this untreated portion of the orbicularis oculi muscle. Botulinum toxin may be directly placed in the superior lateral orbicularis oculi muscle to reduce these wrinkles (see Eyebrow Lift chapter).
  - **Lower eyelid wrinkles** can be due to several different causes, and a stepwise approach may be used to achieve improvement, which is outlined as follows:

- Lower eyelid wrinkles may result from compensatory contraction of the **medial preseptal orbicularis oculi muscle** after treatment of the crow's feet. Reducing the botulinum toxin dose at the third injection point may reduce lower eyelid wrinkles resulting from medial orbicularis oculi contraction.
- If this does not effect enough reduction in lower eyelid wrinkles, botulinum toxin may be placed directly in the **preseptal orbicularis oculi muscle** (see Lower Eyelid Wrinkles chapter).

Complications and Management

- General injection-related complications (see Introduction and Foundation Concepts section, Complications)
- Bruising
- Photophobia
- Lip ptosis with resultant smile asymmetry
- Oral incompetence with resultant drooling and impaired speaking, eating, or drinking
- Blepharoptosis (droopy upper eyelid)
- Diplopia (double vision)
- Lagophthalmos (incomplete eyelid closure)
- Impaired blink reflex
- Ectropion of the lower eyelid (eyelid margin eversion)
- Xerophthalmia (dry eye)
- Globe trauma

Bruising (ecchymosis) is the most common complication seen with treatment of crow's feet. Bruises can range in size from pinpoint needle insertion marks to quarter-sized bruises or hematomas, and if extravasated blood spreads, a "black eye" seen as a large infraocular ecchymotic crescent may occur. The time for resolution of a bruise depends on the patients' physiology and the size of the bruise. Larger bruises can be visible for 1–2 weeks. Prevention of bruising is preferable and several suggestions for bruise prevention are listed in the Introduction and Foundation Concepts section, Preprocedure Checklist. Immediate application of ice and pressure to a bruise can minimize bruising.

Photophobia is uncommon and when it occurs, is usually mild. It typically results from reduced squinting. Using sun protective measures such as sunglasses and hats can alleviate this problem.

Lip and cheek ptosis causing smile asymmetry and/or oral incompetence with resultant drooling and impaired speaking, eating, or drinking can occur with injections placed deeply and inferiorly, below the superior margin of the zygoma. The zygomaticus major lip levator muscle is most frequently involved as it is adjacent to the orbicularis oculi muscle and when affected, typically presents with lip and cheek ptosis similar to Bell's palsy, without oral incompetence. Patients who have undergone facial plastic surgery may be at increased risk of zygomaticus major involvement because of altered periocular anatomy.

Blepharoptosis is uncommon with crow's feet treatments and more commonly seen with frown line treatments. Botulinum toxin placed superiorly can migrate into the levator muscles of the upper eyelid causing blepharoptosis. See Frown Lines chapter, Complications for additional information on blepharoptosis and management strategies.

    Impaired eyelid function and altered lower eyelid position, such as ectropion and lagophthalmos, are very rare and can occur with high botulinum toxin doses which excessively weaken the palpebral orbicularis oculi, or if botulinum toxin is placed too close to the eyelid. **Xerophthalmia,** which is extremely rare, can result from impaired eyelid function with reduced lacrimal flow, or may be secondary to ectropion and lagophthalmos. Patients who have had LASIK surgery may be more susceptible to xerophthalmia. **Diplopia** can occur with deep migration of botulinum toxin into extraocular muscles. **Globe trauma** is a risk with injections placed near the eye. Consultation with an ophthalmologist is advisable with any of these conditions to help in preventing corneal injury and other ocular complications.

Combining Aesthetic Treatments and Maximizing Results

- **Static crow's feet.** Botulinum toxin in the orbicularis oculi muscle can be combined with other minimally invasive aesthetic procedures to enhance static crow's feet results.
    - **Dermal fillers.** Static crow's feet are shown in Figure 7, before (Fig. 7A) and after (Fig. 7B) combination treatment with botulinum toxin in the orbicularis oculi muscle and dermal filler treatment of the zygoma.

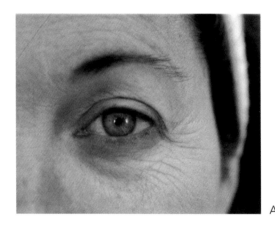

A

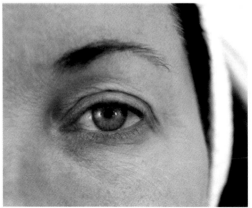

FIGURE 7 ● Static crow's feet before **(A)** and after **(B)** combination treatment with botulinum toxin in the orbicularis oculi muscle and dermal filler treatment of the zygoma. Copyright R. Small, MD.

B

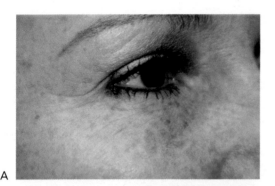

A

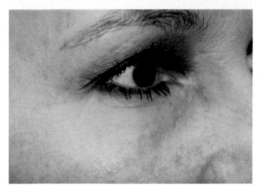

B

FIGURE 8 ● Static crow's feet before
(A) and after **(B)** combination treatment
with botulinum toxin in the orbicularis
oculi muscle and periocular fractional
ablative resurfacing. Copyright
R. Small, MD.

- **Resurfacing procedures,** such as fractional ablative lasers or chemical peels. Static crow's feet are shown in Figure 8, before (Fig. 8A) and after (Fig. 8B) combination treatment with botulinum toxin in the orbicularis oculi muscle and periocular fractional ablative resurfacing.

Pricing

Charges for botulinum toxin treatment of crow's feet range from $200–$500 per treatment or $10–$25 per unit of OBTX.

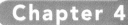

Chapter 4

Lower Eyelid Wrinkles

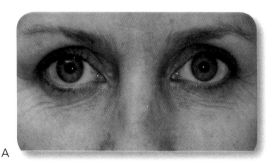
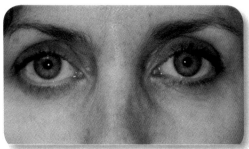

A   B

FIGURE 1 ● Infraocular lines before **(A)** and 1 month after **(B)** botulinum toxin treatment of the inferior orbicularis oculi muscle. Copyright R. Small, MD.

Contraction of the inferior portion of the orbicularis oculi muscle contributes to formation of lower eyelid wrinkles. Treatment of the inferior orbicularis oculi muscle with botulinum toxin focally inhibits contraction, which results in reduction of lower eyelid wrinkles and opening of the eye aperture.

Indications

- Lower eyelid wrinkles
- Palpebral aperture enlargement (i.e., the distance between upper and lower eyelid margins) and rounding of the eye shape
- Lower eyelid muscle bulge, also called a "jelly roll"

Contraindications

- See Introduction and Foundation Concepts section, Contraindications.
- Severe lower eyelid dermatochalasis (skin laxity).
- Abnormal snap test.
- Prominent infraorbital festoons (eye bags).

55

- Lagophthalmos (incomplete closure of eyelids).
- Excessive lower eyelid scleral show.
- Ectropion (eversion of eyelid margin).

It is advisable to use caution in patients who have had previous lower eyelid surgery (e.g., blepharoplasty) or aggressive lower eyelid resurfacing (e.g., ablative laser resurfacing or deeper chemical peels) as they may exhibit lagophthalmos, excessive lower eyelid scleral show, or an ectropion, which contraindicate treatment with botulinum toxin.

Anatomy

- **Wrinkles.** Lower eyelid wrinkles, or infraocular rhytids, course horizontally and radiate inferior laterally away from the lower eyelid (Fig. 1A and 2B). They are often associated with a lower eyelid muscle bulge seen with animation, referred to as a "jelly roll" (Fig. 2A). Lower eyelid wrinkles occur with facial expressions and may be accentuated by botulinum toxin treatment of the crow's feet.
- **Muscles targeted.** Lower eyelid wrinkle treatments with botulinum toxin target the preseptal orbicularis oculi muscle. The orbicularis oculi muscle has an orbital portion which surrounds the eye and a palpebral portion which covers the eye. The palpebral portion is further divided into the preseptal fibers, which course in front of the orbital septum, and the pretarsal fibers, which form the eyelids (Fig. 3).

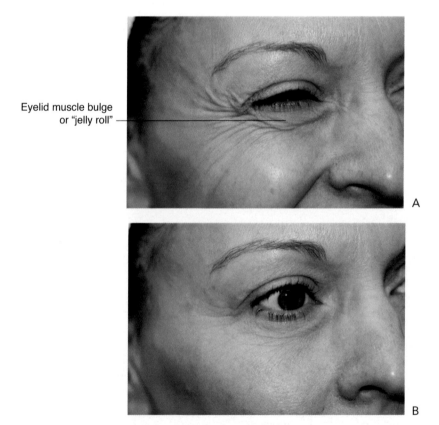

Eyelid muscle bulge or "jelly roll"

A

B

FIGURE 2 ● Lower eyelid dynamic wrinkles and muscle bulge **(A)** and static wrinkles **(B)**. Copyright R. Small, MD.

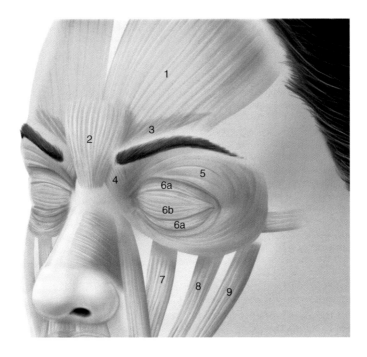

1. Frontalis m.   6. Orbicularis oculi m. (palpebral portion)
2. Procerus m.   a. Preseptal
3. Corrugator supercilii m.   b. Pretarsal
4. Depressor supercilli m.   7. Levator labii superioris m.
5. Orbicularis oculi m. (orbital portion) 8. Zygomaticus minor m.
                                         9. Zygomaticus major m.

FIGURE 3 ● Periocular detailed anatomy. Copyright R. Small, MD.

- **Muscle functions.** Contraction of several different muscles and muscle regions can contribute to formation of lower eyelid wrinkles including the: preseptal orbicularis oculi medial to the mid pupilary line, preseptal orbicularis oculi lateral to the mid pupilary line, and lip levators such as zygomaticus major and levator labii superioris which primarily functions as a lip levator. A lower eyelid muscle bulge is due to contraction of the palpebral portion of the orbicularis muscle.

Patient Assessment

- **Facial surgery** history is obtained, including blepharoplasty and skin resurfacing procedures such as ablative laser resurfacing or deep chemical peels of the lower eyelids. Ophthalmologic history including keratorefractive surgery (LASIK) is obtained as these patients may have a greater risk of dry eyes.
- **Dynamic** (with muscle contraction) assessments of the lower eyelid are made including:
  - **Lower eyelid wrinkles** are evaluated while having the patient perform one of the facial expressions listed below (Fig. 2A). The botulinum toxin injection techniques described in this chapter can reduce lower eyelid wrinkles at or lateral to the mid pupilary line. They do not reduce lower eyelid wrinkles medial to the mid pupilary line.
  - **Lower eyelid wrinkles muscle bulge** is also assessed while the patient is contracting the lower eyelid muscles (Fig. 2A). Botulinum toxin injection of the lower

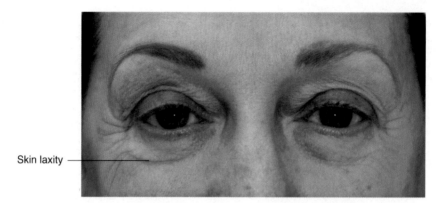

Skin laxity

FIGURE 4 ● Laxity of the lower eyelid is a contraindication to botulinum toxin treatment of the lower eyelid. Copyright R. Small, MD.

eyelid can soften this muscle bulge and increase the palpebral aperture, which can widen and round the eye shape.

- **Static** (at rest) assessments of the lower eyelid are made including:
  - **Static lower eyelid wrinkles** are assessed with the face at rest (Fig. 2B).
  - **Skin laxity** of the lower eyelids may be clinically evident as wrinkles and folds of skin in the lower eyelid area (Fig. 4). Botulinum toxin treatment of the lower eyelid may exacerbate these wrinkles and treatment should be avoided in patients with obvious skin laxity. Surgery is often required to improve lower eyelid wrinkles due to severe skin laxity.
  - **Elasticity of the lower eyelids** is assessed using the **snap test**. It is performed by grasping the skin of the lower eyelid between the thumb and the first finger, pulling the skin gently away from the eye and releasing (Fig. 5). If the skin recoils immediately, the snap test is normal and botulinum toxin treatment may be performed. If the skin recoils slowly (more than 3 seconds), the lower eyelid has insufficient elasticity and should not be treated with botulinum toxin.

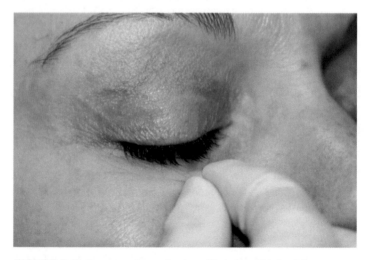

FIGURE 5 ● Snap test for evaluation of lower eyelid elasticity. Copyright R. Small, MD.

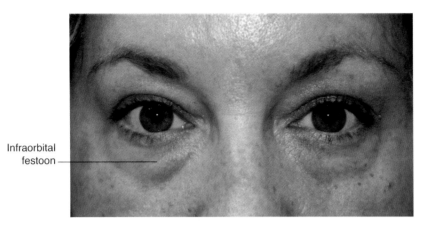

Infraorbital
festoon

FIGURE 6 ● Infraorbital festoons are a contraindication to botulinum toxin treatment
of the lower eyelids. Copyright R. Small, MD.

- **Infraorbital festoons,** or lower eye bags, are soft tissue bulges, which are visible at rest (Fig. 6). The orbital septum, which is a facial layer that helps to retain infraorbital fat pads, weakens with age. Eye bags are typically due to bulging of the infraorbital fat pad as a result of a weakened orbital septum. The orbicularis oculi also supports the inferior orbital septum and weakening of this muscle with botulinum toxin may exacerbate festooning. Treatment should be avoided in patients with eye bags.
- **Scleral show** refers to the crescent of white sclera visible between the iris and the lower eyelid margin at rest with forward level gaze. Scleral show is due to lower lid retraction and, while a small amount of sclera show is common and a normal finding, excessive sclera show of more than 2 mm is a contraindication to botulinum toxin treatment of the lower eyelid.
- **Lagophthalmos** is incomplete closure of eyelids and can be assessed by instructing the patient to "roll their eyes upwards" while trying to keep their eyelids closed. Figure 7 shows a patient with a history of a blepharoplasty demonstrating lagophthalmos with upward gaze. This is a contraindication to botulinum toxin treatment of the lower eyelids.

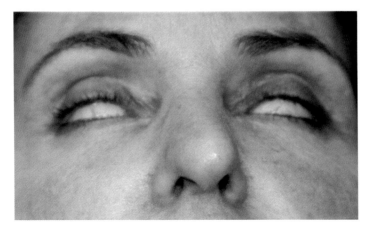

FIGURE 7 ● Incomplete eyelid closure (lagophthalmos), shown in a
patient with a history of a blepharoplasty, is a contraindication to botulinum toxin treatment of the lower eyelids. Copyright R. Small, MD.

Eliciting Contraction of Muscles to Be Treated

Instruct the patient to perform any of the following expressions:

- "Make a cheesy grin" or "make a big smile"
- "Squint like the sun is in your eyes"

Treatment Goal

- Partial inhibition of the inferior orbicularis oculi muscle.

Reconstitution

- Reconstitute 100 units of Botox Cosmetic powder with 4 mL of nonpreserved sterile saline (see Introduction and Foundation Concepts section, Reconstitution Method).
- Botulinum toxin products are not interchangeable and all references in this chapter to onabotulinumtoxinA (OBTX) refer specifically to Botox.

Starting Doses

- Women and men: total (bilateral) dose is 2.5 units of OBTX

Anesthesia

- Anesthesia with ice is not recommended because it vasoconstricts and can obscure blood vessels.

Equipment for Treatment

- General botulinum toxin supplies (see Introduction and Foundation Concepts section, Equipment)
- Reconstituted Botox Cosmetic
- 30- or 32-gauge 0.5-inch needle

Procedure Overview

- An overview of injection points and OBTX doses for treatment of lower eyelid wrinkles is shown in Figure 8. Two injections are usually performed for each eye, one medial (Fig. 8A) and one lateral (Fig. 8B). Providers getting started with botulinum toxin injections may choose to start with injection of the medial point only (Fig. 8A), to reduce the risk of complications.
- Botulinum toxin is injected subdermally for treatment of lower eyelid wrinkles. These injections require a light touch as the orbicularis oculi muscle is a superficial muscle and the lower eyelid skin is very thin.
- For patients with long eyelashes that obscure the medial injection point instruct them to "roll their eyes upward" while keeping their eyelids closed when performing this injection.
- The inferior eyelid region has many tiny veins, which are best seen and avoided using oblique lighting.

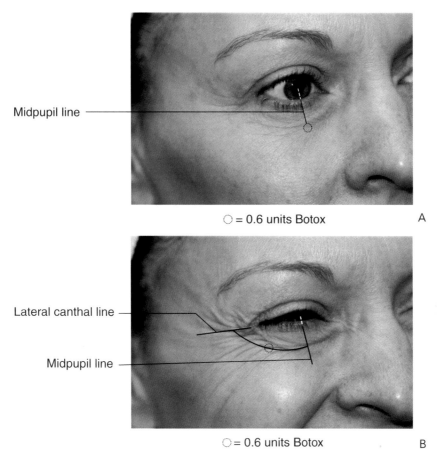

Midpupil line

◌ = 0.6 units Botox   A

Lateral canthal line

Midpupil line

◌ = 0.6 units Botox   B

FIGURE 8 ● Overview of botulinum toxin injection points and doses for treatment of lower eyelid wrinkles. The medial injection is placed with the muscles at rest **(A)** and the lateral injection is placed during orbicularis oculi muscle contraction **(B)**. Copyright R. Small, MD.

- Injecting superiorly may involve the pretarsal orbicularis oculi muscle and increase the risk of lower eyelid ectropion and lagophthalmos.

Technique

1. Position the patient at a 60-degree reclined position.
2. Identify facial landmarks. Palpate the orbital rim (Fig. 9). Identify the lateral canthal and midpupillary lines (Fig. 8).
3. Prepare injection sites with alcohol and allow them to dry.
4. The provider is positioned on the side that is to be injected.
5. **Medial lower eyelid injection**. The medial lower eyelid injection is located in the midpupillary line, 0.5 cm inferior to the eyelid margin (Fig. 8A). While the muscles are at rest and patient's eyes are closed, angle the needle medially, almost parallel to the skin, and insert the needle tip subdermally just under the skin. Inject 0.6 units of OBTX to raise a wheal (Fig. 10).
6. **Lateral lower eyelid injection**. The lateral lower eyelid injection point is located midway between the first injection point and the lateral canthal line, 1 cm inferior to

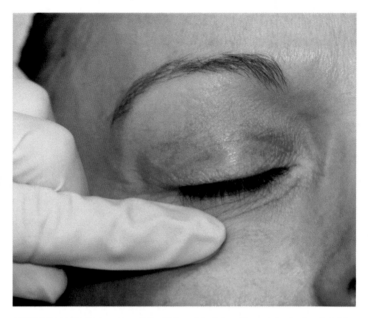

FIGURE 9 ● Palpation of the infraorbital rim. Copyright R. Small, MD.

the eyelid margin (Fig. 8B). While the orbicularis oculi muscle contracted, angle the needle inferiorly, almost parallel to the skin, and insert the needle tip subdermally just under the skin. Inject 0.6 units of OBTX to raise a wheal (Fig. 11).

7. Repeat injections for the contralateral inferior orbicularis oculi muscle.
8. Compress the injection sites, directing pressure away from the eye.

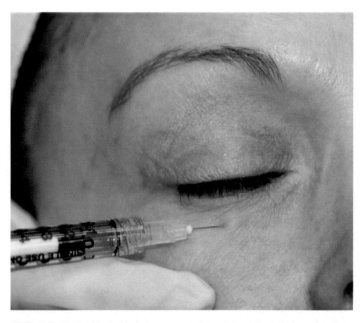

FIGURE 10 ● Medial botulinum toxin injection of the inferior orbicularis oculi muscle. Copyright R. Small, MD.

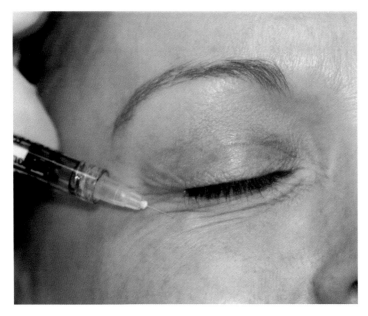

FIGURE 11 ● Lateral botulinum toxin injection of the inferior orbicularis oculi muscle. Copyright R. Small, MD.

Results

- **Reduction of lower eyelid wrinkles, "jelly rolls"**, and **eye aperture enlargement** are typically seen 3 days after botulinum toxin treatment, with maximal improvements at 1–2 weeks (Figs. 1A and 1B). Unlike with botulinum toxin treatments in other regions of the face, both static and dynamic lower eyelid wrinkles usually respond well to treatment.

Duration of Effects and Treatment Intervals

- Muscle function in the treatment area gradually returns 2.5–3 months after botulinum toxin treatment.
- Subsequent lower eyelid treatments with botulinum toxin may be performed when the orbicularis oculi muscle begins to contract, before lines and wrinkles return to their pretreatment appearance.

Follow-Ups and Management

Patients are assessed 2 weeks after botulinum toxin treatment to evaluate for reduction of lower eyelid wrinkles and eyelid position. Persistent lower eyelid wrinkles are often due to one of the following reasons:

- **Deep static wrinkling.** If static wrinkles are present, patients may require several consecutive botulinum toxin treatments for results to be seen. Botulinum toxin doses are not routinely escalated in the lower eyelid region because of the increased risk of complications with higher doses. Combining botulinum toxin with other minimally invasive aesthetic procedures can offer enhanced results for treatment of static lower eyelid wrinkles (see Combining Aesthetic Treatments on next page).

- **Adjacent muscle involvement.** In some patients, lower eyelid wrinkles result from upward movement of the cheek due to contraction of the zygomaticus and/or levator labii superioris muscles. These patients will not benefit from botulinum toxin treatment of the lower eyelid.

Complications and Management

- General Injection-Related Complications (see Introduction and Foundation Concepts, Complications)
- Worsening infraocular festooning (eye bags)
- Lagophthalmos (incomplete eyelid closure)
- Impaired blink reflex
- Ectropion of the lower eyelid (eyelid margin eversion)
- Xerophthalmia (dry eyes)
- Globe trauma
- Epiphora (tearing)

Infraocular festoons may worsen due to botulinum toxin injection in the lower eyelid area due to weakening of the inferior orbicularis oculi muscle and/or impaired lymphatic drainage.

Impaired eyelid function and **altered eyelid position,** such as **ectropion** and **lagophthalmos,** are very rare and can occur with high botulinum toxin doses excessively weakening the palpebral orbicularis oculi or if botulinum toxin is placed too close to the eyelid. One study (Flynn, 2003) suggests that botulinum toxin placed in the lateral palpebral orbicularis oculi muscle injection point described earlier, may be associated with an increased risk of ectropion.

Xerophthalmia, which is extremely rare, can result from impaired eyelid function with reduced lacrimal flow or may be secondary to ectropion and lagophthalmos. Patients who have had LASIK surgery may be more susceptible to xerophthalmia. **Epiphora** may result from lacrimal dysfunction, if botulinum toxin is placed medial to the midpupillary line. **Globe trauma** is a risk as injections in the lower eyelid area are usually superior to the bony orbital rim.

There are no corrective treatments for most of these complications; however, they will spontaneously resolve as botulinum toxin effects diminish. Consultation with an ophthalmologist is advisable with any of these complications.

Combining Aesthetic Treatments and Maximizing Results

- **Static lower eyelid wrinkles.** Combination therapy with resurfacing procedures such as fractional ablative lasers or chemical peels, together with botulinum toxin in the inferior orbicularis oculi muscle, can enhance static lower eyelid wrinkle results.

Pricing

Treatment of lower eyelid wrinkles is typically performed concomitantly with treatment of the crow's feet. This is an advanced botulinum toxin treatment area and charges range from $50–$60 per unit of OBTX.

Chapter 5

Eyebrow Lift

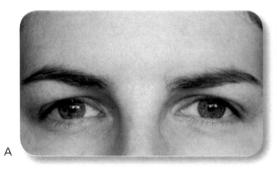 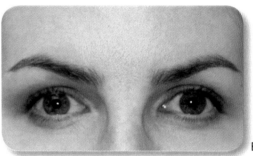

A   B

FIGURE 1 ● Eyebrow lift before **(A)** and 2 weeks after **(B)** botulinum toxin treatment of the infrabrow orbicularis oculi muscle in a patient also receiving botulinum toxin treatment of the glabellar complex muscles for frown line treatment, at rest. Copyright R. Small, MD.

Low-positioned eyebrows (eyebrow ptosis) and upper eyelid skin laxity (dermatochalasis) convey a tired or sad appearance and are accentuated by contraction of the superior lateral orbicularis oculi muscle. These conditions can often be improved with botulinum toxin treatment of the superior lateral orbicularis oculi which inhibits muscle contraction resulting in lateral eyebrow elevation, also called a chemical brow lift or eyebrow lift. Treatment of other muscle groups in the upper face can also elevate eyebrows (see Combining Aesthetic Treatments at the end of this chapter), however, botulinum toxin treatment of the superior lateral orbicularis oculi muscle is the focus of this chapter.

Indications

- Lateral eyebrow ptosis
- Upper eyelid dermatochalasis
- Lateral eyebrow lift

Anatomy

- **Eyebrow position and shape.** In women, ideal eyebrow position is slightly above the supraorbital ridge and that the brow has an arched, tapering gull-wing shape (Fig. 2A).

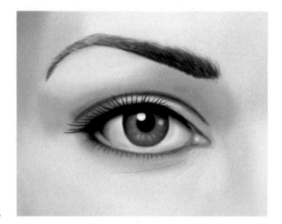

A

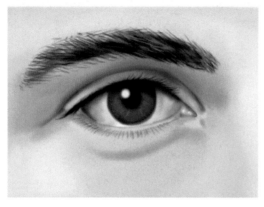

B

FIGURE 2 ● Eyebrow shapes: women **(A)** and men **(B)**. Copyright R. Small, MD.

In men, eyebrows are positioned at the supraorbital ridge and are horizontal in shape (Fig. 2B).

- **Muscles targeted.** Lateral eyebrow lift with botulinum toxin targets the superior lateral orbital portion of the orbicularis oculi muscle. Other muscles in the upper face affecting eyebrow height position and are listed in Table 1.

TABLE 1

Eyebrow Height and Position: Effects of Muscle Contraction and Botulinum Toxin Treatments

Muscle	Muscle Contraction Effect on Eyebrow	Botulinum Toxin Effect on Eyebrow
Glabellar complex	Medial eyebrow depressor	Elevates medial eyebrow
Superior lateral orbicularis oculi	Lateral eyebrow depressor	Elevates lateral eyebrow
Lateral orbicularis oculi	Lateral eyebrow depressor	Elevates lateral eyebrow
Frontalis	Medial and lateral eyebrow levator	Lowers medial and lateral eyebrow

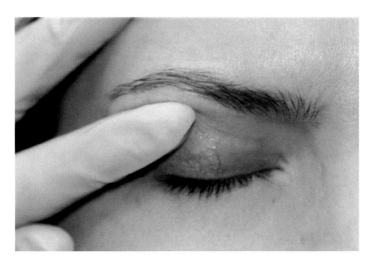

FIGURE 3 ● Superior lateral orbicularis muscle targeted with botulinum toxin eyebrow lift treatments. Copyright R. Small, MD.

- **Muscle functions.** Contraction of the superior lateral orbicularis oculi muscle lowers the lateral eyebrow, and aids in closure of the eyelid and lacrimal function (see Anatomy section, Figs. 1 and 2).

Patient Assessment

- **Eyebrow ptosis** and **dermatochalasis** (hooding) are assessed with the frontalis muscle at rest. Patients with severe dermatochalasis who have excessive folds of lax skin resting on the upper eyelid, or significant eyebrow ptosis, typically do not show marked improvement with lateral eyebrow lifting and may require surgical interventions such as blepharoplasty and a forehead lift, respectively.
- **Strength of the superior lateral orbicularis oculi muscle** is assessed by placing the index finger beneath this portion of the muscle and having the patient contract the muscle (Fig. 3). If the patient can exert forceful pressure against the finger with a visible roll of contracted muscle, the eyebrow lift procedure will typically yield noticeable elevation of the lateral eyebrow.

Eliciting Contraction of the Muscles to Be Treated

Instruct the patient to perform the following expression:

- "Blink hard and hold it"

Treatment Goal

- Partial inhibition of the superior lateral orbicularis oculi muscle.

Reconstitution

- Reconstitute 100 units of Botox Cosmetic powder with 4 mL of nonpreserved saline (see Introduction and Foundation Concepts section, Reconstitution Method).

- Botulinum toxin products are not interchangeable and all references in this chapter to onabotulinumtoxinA (OBTX) refer specifically to Botox.

Starting Doses

- Women: total (bilateral) dose is 5–7.5 units of OBTX.
- Men: total (bilateral) dose is 7.5–10 units of OBTX.

Anesthesia

- Anesthesia is not necessary for most patients but an ice pack may be used if required.

Equipment for Treatment

- General botulinum toxin injection supplies (see Introduction and Foundation Concepts section, Equipment)
- Reconstituted Botox Cosmetic
- 30-gauge, 0.5-inch needle

Procedure Overview

- Place injections in the eyebrow lift safety zone (Fig. 4). The safety zone is at least 1 cm outside the orbital rim, below the supraorbital ridge and lateral to the lateral limbus line.
- An overview of injection points and OBTX doses for a lateral eyebrow lift is shown in Figure 5.
- Botulinum toxin is injected intramuscularly with the eyebrow lift procedure.
- Injecting superior lateral to the safety zone may involve the frontalis muscle, resulting in eyebrow ptosis.
- Injecting superior medial to the safety zone at the lateral limbus line may involve eyelid levator muscles, resulting in blepharoptosis (droopy upper eyelid).

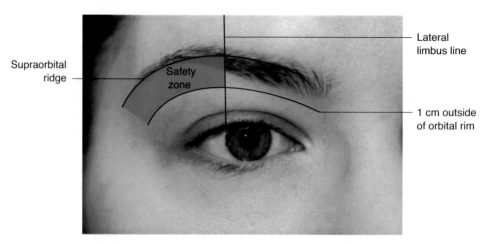

FIGURE 4 ● Eyebrow lift safety zone for botulinum toxin treatments. Copyright R. Small, MD.

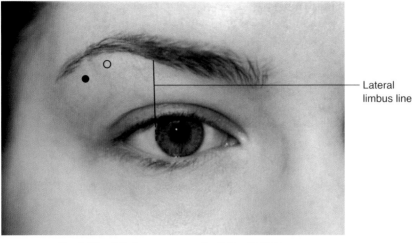

O = 1.25 unit Botox   ● = 2.5 units Botox

FIGURE 5 ● Overview of botulinum toxin injection points and doses for lateral eye-brow lift. Copyright R. Small, MD.

Technique

1. Position the patient at a 60-degree reclined position.
2. Identify the eyebrow lift safety zone (Fig. 4).
3. Identify the superior lateral portion of the orbicularis oculi muscle by instructing the patient to contract the muscle as described above and visualizing/palpating the roll of contracted muscle (Fig. 3).
4. Identify the injection points (Fig. 5).
5. Ice for anesthesia (optional).
6. Prepare injection sites with alcohol and allow to dry.
7. The provider is positioned on the side that is to be injected.

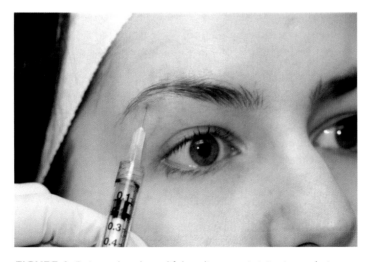

FIGURE 6 ● Lateral eyebrow lift botulinum toxin injection technique. Copyright R. Small, MD.

8. While the orbicularis oculi muscle is relaxed, insert the needle in the first injection point located approximately 1.5 cm lateral to the lateral limbus line, within the safety zone (Fig. 6). Angle the needle towards the forehead and insert subdermally. Inject 2.5 units of OBTX.
9. The second injection point is 1 cm medial to the first injection point, closer to the lateral limbus line. Insert the needle similarly and inject 1.25 units of OBTX.
10. Repeat the above injections for the contralateral side of the face.
11. Compress the injection sites firmly, directing pressure away from the eye.

Results

- **Lateral eyebrow elevation** is typically noticeable 1–2 weeks after botulinum toxin treatment (Figs. 1A and 1B).

Duration of Effects and Treatment Intervals

- Muscle function in the treatment area gradually returns 2–3 months after botulinum toxin treatment.
- Eyebrow lifting is subtle and determining when to return for treatment can be challenging for patients. Subsequent treatments may be performed when eyebrow descent is noticeable or when patients notice recurrence of eyelid heaviness or a fatigued appearance. The author typically performs an eyebrow lift every 3–4 months with the same time intervals as other upper face botulinum toxin treatments.

Follow-Ups and Management

Patients are assessed 2 weeks after botulinum toxin treatment to evaluate for reduction of eyebrow ptosis. If more lateral eyebrow elevation is desired, assess the strength of the superior lateral orbicularis oculi muscle. If significant contractility is still present, additional OBTX may be injected in the same areas previously treated. Total bilateral doses for this touch-up procedure are usually 2.5–5 units of OBTX.

Complications and Management

- General injection-related complications (see Botulinum Toxin Introduction and Foundation Concepts section, Complications topic)
- Blepharoptosis

   Blepharoptosis may occur as a complication from eyebrow lift treatments, particularly if botulinum toxin is injected too close to the supraorbital ridge at the lateral limbus line. Blepharoptosis results from migration of botulinum toxin through the orbital septum fascia to the levator palpebrae superioris muscle in the upper eyelid (See Frown Lines chapter for treatment of blepharoptosis).

Combining Aesthetic Treatments and Maximizing Results

Eyebrow position and height can be optimized by combining a lateral eyebrow lift with the following procedures:

- **Botulinum toxin.** Treatments in other muscles of the upper face can enhance eyebrow elevation, including:
  - Glabellar complex muscles (see Frown Lines chapter) for additional medial eyebrow elevation.
  - Lateral orbicularis oculi muscle (see Crow's Feet chapter) for additional lateral eyebrow elevation.
  - Frontalis muscle, using the "V-shaped" injection pattern (see Horizontal Forehead Lines chapter) for additional lateral eyebrow elevation.
- **Dermal fillers.** Lateral eyebrow elevation can also be augmented by combining botulinum toxin lateral eyebrow lift with infrabrow dermal filler treatments.

Pricing

Charges for botulinum toxin eyebrow lift treatments range from $150–$200 per treatment or $10–$25 per unit of OBTX.

Chapter 6

Bunny Lines

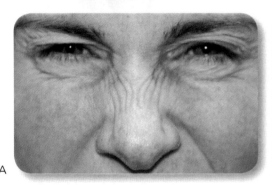 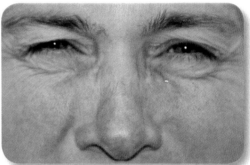

A   B

FIGURE 1 ● Bunny lines before **(A)** and 2 weeks after **(B)** botulinum toxin treatment of the nasalis muscle, with active nasal scrunching. Copyright R. Small, MD.

Dynamic bunny lines result from contraction of the nasalis muscle. They are part of facial expressions such as frowning, squinting, or smiling and may also be accentuated by botulinum toxin treatments in the upper face for frown lines and crow's feet. Botulinum toxin treatment of the nasalis reduces bunny lines by inhibiting muscle contraction and smoothing the overlying skin.

Indication

- Bunny lines

Anatomy

- **Wrinkles.** Bunny lines, or nasalis rhytids, are wrinkles formed on the lateral and dorsal aspects of the nose. They typically course diagonally over the nasal sidewalls and nasal bridge (Fig. 1A and see Anatomy section, Figs. 4 and 5). Transverse lines across the root of the nose are not related to the nasalis muscle but rather are due to contraction of the procerus muscle seen with frowning (Fig. 2).
- **Muscles targeted.** Botulinum toxin bunny line treatment targets the nasalis muscle (see Anatomy section, Figs. 1 and 2).

73

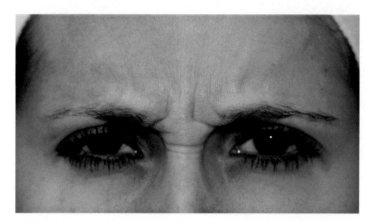

FIGURE 2 ● Transverse nasal lines due to contraction of the procerus muscle. Copyright R. Small, MD.

- **Muscle functions.** Nasalis contraction draws the nasal sidewalls superiorly and medially, producing bunny lines (see Anatomy section, Fig. 7). In some individuals this also leads to fine medial infraocular lines.
- **Muscles avoided.** The levator labii superioris alaeque nasi muscle that lies on the lateral border of the nasalis muscle can also contribute to formation of bunny lines. This is primarily an upper lip levator and, as with other lip levators, it is avoided with treatment of bunny lines. Other upper lip levator muscles that are avoided with botulinum toxin treatment of bunny lines include, in order of medial to lateral location, levator labii superioris, zygomaticus minor, and zygomaticus major (see Anatomy section, Fig. 3).

Patient Assessment

- **Dynamic** (with muscle contraction) and **static** (at rest) **bunny lines** are assessed.
- **Concomitant contraction of the nasalis, glabellar and/or orbicularis oculi muscles** during facial animation are assessed. Patients that form bunny lines with these other facial expressions will benefit from botulinum toxin treatment of bunny lines concomitantly with these other facial areas.

Eliciting Contraction of Muscles to Be Treated

Instruct the patient to perform the following expression:

- "Think of a bad skunk smell"

Treatment Goal

- Complete inhibition of the nasalis muscle.

Reconstitution

- Reconstitute 100 units of Botox Cosmetic powder with 4 mL of nonpreserved saline (see Introduction and Foundation Concepts section, Reconstitution Method).

- Botulinum toxin products are not interchangeable and all references in this chapter to onabotulinumtoxinA (OBTX) refer specifically to Botox.

Starting Doses

- Women and men: 2.5–5 units of OBTX

Anesthesia

- Anesthesia is not necessary for most patients but an ice pack may be used if required.

Equipment for Treatment

- General botulinum toxin injection supplies (see Introduction and Foundation Concepts section, Equipment)
- Reconstituted Botox Cosmetic
- 30-gauge, 0.5-inch needle

Procedure Overview

- Place injections within the bunny line safety zone (Figs. 3A and 3B). The safety zone is a diamond-shaped region with the superior point of the diamond located at the nasion (the least protruding part of the nose between the medial canthi) and the inferior point located halfway between the nasion and nasal tip. The lateral diamond points lie along the nasion-ala line. The nasion-ala line is drawn from the edge of the nasal ala inferiorly and intersects the intercanthal line superiorly.
- An overview of injection points and OBTX doses for treatment of bunny lines is shown in Figure 4.
- Botulinum toxin is injected intramuscularly for treatment of bunny lines.
- Injecting lateral to the safety zone may involve the labii superioris alaeque nasi muscle, resulting in upper lip ptosis (droopy upper lip).
- Injecting superior lateral to the safety zone may involve the medial palpebral orbicularis oculi, which can disrupt lacrimal drainage resulting in epiphoria (excessive tearing).
- Injecting superior to the safety zone may involve the procerus muscle and does not target the nasalis muscle.

Technique

1. Position the patient at a 60-degree reclined position.
2. Identify the bunny line safety zone (Fig. 3).
3. Locate the nasalis muscles by instructing the patient to contract the muscles using one of the facial expression above.
4. Identify the injection points (Fig. 4).
5. Ice for anesthesia (optional).
6. Prepare injection sites with alcohol and allow to dry.
7. The provider is positioned on the side that is to be injected.
8. While the nasalis muscle is contracted, insert the needle just medial to the nasion-ala line located on the lateral nasal wall within the safety zone (Fig. 5). Angle

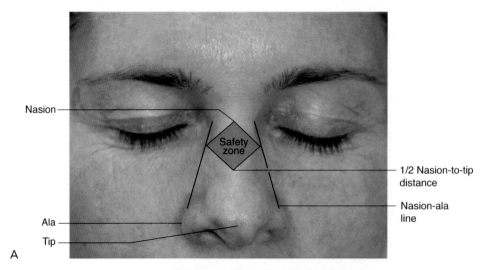

A

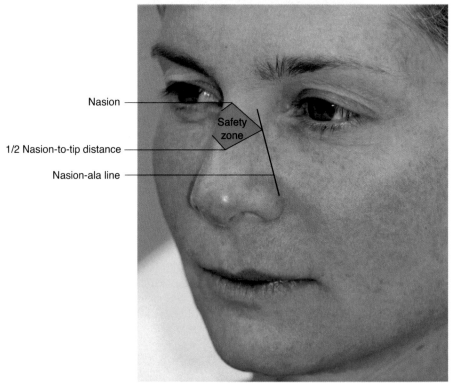

B

FIGURE 3 ● Bunny line safety zone for botulinum toxin treatments: anterior-posterior **(A)** and oblique **(B)** views. Copyright R. Small, MD.

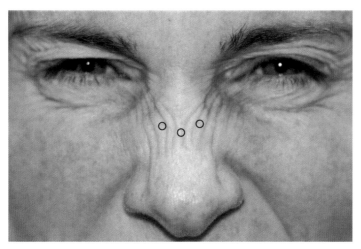

O = 1.25 units Botox

FIGURE 4 ● Overview of botulinum toxin injection points and doses for treatment of bunny lines. Copyright R. Small, MD.

the needle towards the nasal sidewall and insert subdermally. Inject 1.25 units of OBTX.

9. Repeat the above injection on the contralateral nasal wall.

10. The third injection point is on the dorsum of the nose. Reposition to stand in front of the patient. With the nasalis muscle contracted, approach inferiorly,

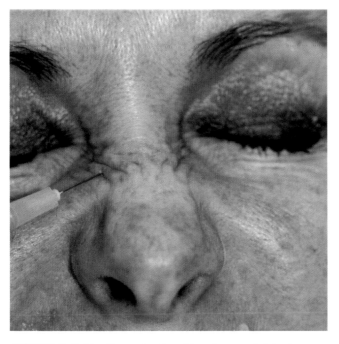

FIGURE 5 ● Nasalis muscle sidewall botulinum toxin injection technique. Copyright R. Small, MD.

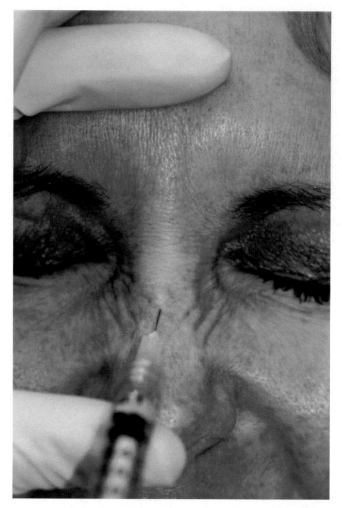

FIGURE 6 ● Nasalis muscle dorsum botulinum toxin injection technique. Copyright R. Small, MD.

angling the needle toward the dorsum of the nose, and inject 1.25 units of OBTX (Fig. 6).

11. Compress injection wheals medially.

Results

- **Reduction of dynamic bunny lines** is typically seen 3 days after botulinum toxin treatment, with maximal reduction at 2 weeks (Figs. 1A and 1B).

Duration of Effects and Treatment Intervals

- Muscle function in the treatment area gradually returns 3–4 months after botulinum toxin treatment.

- Subsequent bunny line treatments with botulinum toxin may be performed when the nasalis muscle begins to contract, before the lines return to their pretreatment appearance.

Follow-Ups and Management

Patients are assessed 2 weeks after botulinum toxin treatment to evaluate for reduced bunny lines. If persistent bunny lines are present, evaluate for one of the following common causes:

- **Persistent nasalis muscle contraction.** Some patients may have greater muscle mass than anticipated in the treatment area and additional botulinum toxin may be required to achieve desired results. Persistent muscle contraction can be corrected with a touch-up procedure using 1.25–2.5 units of OBTX, depending on the degree of nasalis muscle activity present.
- **Static lines.** If static lines are present, patients may require several consecutive treatments for results to be seen.

Complications and Management

- General injection-related complications (see Introduction and Foundation Concepts section, Complications)
- Lip ptosis with resultant smile asymmetry
- Oral incompetence with resultant drooling and impaired speaking, eating, or drinking
- Epiphoria
- Diplopia

Most complications with bunny line treatments occur if injections are placed laterally along the nasal sidewall, such that botulinum toxin affects the lip levator muscles. These complications can range from mild **lip ptosis** and **smile asymmetry** due to involvement of the levator labii superioris alaeque nasi, to more serious functional impairments resulting from **oral incompetence** such as drooling, impaired speech, and difficulty eating or drinking, due to involvement of zygomaticus and levator labii superioris lip levator muscles.

Epiphoria can result from impaired lacrimal drainage if the medial palpebral portion of the orbicularis oculi is affected. With injections near the lateral canthus, diffusion to extraocular muscles can result in **diplopia.**

There are no corrective treatments for most of these complications; however, they will spontaneously resolve as botulinum toxin effects diminish. With any of these conditions, consultation with an ophthalmologist is advisable to help prevent corneal injury and other ocular complications.

Combining Aesthetic Treatments and Maximizing Results

- Treatment of bunny lines is often performed concomitantly with botulinum toxin treatment of frown lines or crow's feet (see Frown Lines and Crow's Feet chapters).

Pricing

Charges for botulinum toxin treatment of bunny lines range from $150–$200 per treatment or $10–$25 per unit of OBTX.

Chapter 7

Lip Lines

FIGURE 1 ● Upper lip lines before **(A)** and 2 weeks after **(B)** botulinum toxin treatment of the upper orbicularis oris muscle, with active muscle contraction. Copyright R. Small, MD.

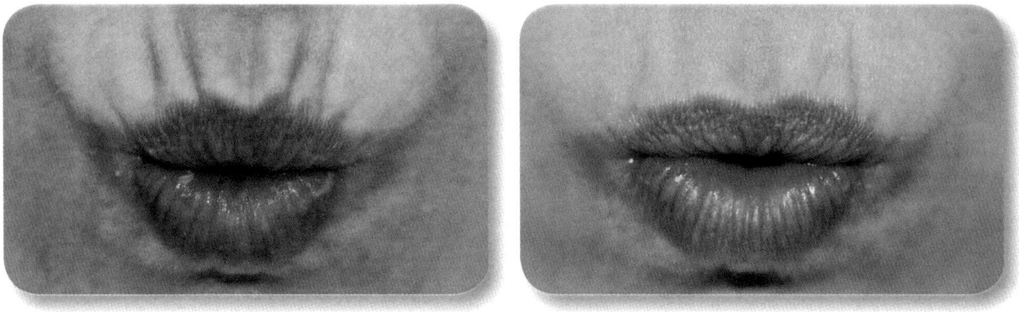

Dynamic lip lines result from contraction of the perioral musculature, primarily the orbicularis oris muscle. Botulinum toxin treatment of the orbicularis oris reduces lip lines by inhibiting muscle contraction and smoothing the overlying skin. Treatment of the orbicularis oculi muscle also increases lip eversion resulting in a fuller lip appearance. Upper lip lines are a common complaint and, while safety zones and injection points for both upper and lower lips are discussed, the focus of this chapter is botulinum toxin treatment of the upper lip.

Indications

- Radial lip lines
- Enhanced lip fullness

Anatomy

- **Wrinkles.** Lip lines, medically referred to as perioral rhytids and commonly referred to as lipstick lines or smoker's lines, are wrinkles that extend radially from the upper and lower lip borders (see Anatomy section, Figs. 4 and 5).

81

- **Muscles targeted.** Botulinum toxin lip line treatment targets the orbicularis oris, a sphincteric muscle that encircles the mouth.
- **Muscle functions.** The orbicularis oris muscle functions to draw the lips medially and to invert the lip border (see Anatomy section, Fig. 7 and Table 1). Adequate strength of the orbicularis oris muscle is required for facial expressions such as smiling and puckering as well as the essential functions of speaking, kissing, eating, and drinking.
- **Muscles avoided.** Many muscles of the middle and lower face insert and exert effects on the lips and most of these muscles lie deep to the orbicularis oris muscle. Upper lip levator muscles avoided with botulinum toxin treatment of lip lines include: levator labii superioris alaeque nasi, levator labii superioris, zygomaticus minor, zygomaticus major, and levator anguli oris (see Anatomy section, Fig. 3).

Patient Assessment

- **Social history** is obtained including occupations/activities necessitating full oral competence, such as wind instrument musicians, actors, singers, and public speakers.
- **Dynamic** (with muscle contraction) and **static** (at rest) **lip lines** are assessed.

Eliciting Contraction of Muscles to Be Treated

Instruct the patient to perform any of the following expressions:

- "Whistle"
- "Sip on a straw"
- "Pucker"

Treatment Goal

- Partial inhibition of the upper lip orbicularis oris muscle to reduce lip lines with avoidance of the philtral area to maintain a desirable lip shape.

Reconstitution

- Reconstitute 100 units of Botox Cosmetic powder with 4 mL of nonpreserved saline (see Introduction and Foundation Concepts section, Reconstitution Method).
- Botulinum toxin products are not interchangeable and all references in this chapter to onabotulinumtoxinA (OBTX) refer specifically to Botox.

Starting Doses

- Women and men: total (bilateral) dose is 3.75–5 units of OBTX for the upper lip

Anesthesia

- The upper lip is very sensitive and anesthesia is required. Topical anesthetics reduce motor function in the applied area, and therefore, are applied after evaluating the area for dynamic wrinkling and taking photographs.

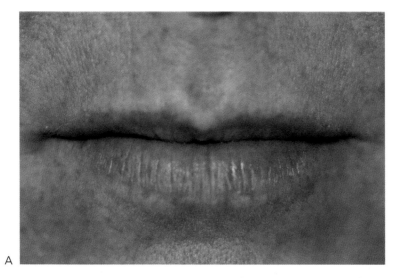

A

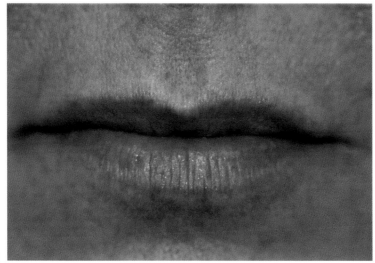

B

FIGURE 2 ● Upper lip fullness before **(A)** and 2 weeks after **(B)** botulinum toxin treatment of the upper orbicularis oris muscle, at rest. Copyright R. Small, MD.

- Apply a topical anesthetic such as benzocaine/lidocaine/tetracaine without occlusion, for 15 minutes before treatment.
- In addition, application of ice to patient tolerance, for up to 1–2 minutes, immediately before treatment is also recommended.

Equipment for Treatment

- General botulinum toxin injection supplies (see Introduction and Foundation Concepts section, Equipment)
- Reconstituted Botox Cosmetic
- 30-gauge, 0.5-inch needle

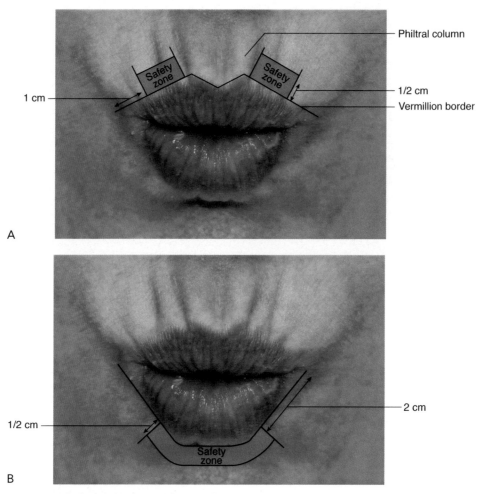

FIGURE 3 ● Lip line safety zones for the upper lip **(A)** and lower lip **(B)**, with botulinum toxin treatments. Copyright R. Small, MD.

Procedure Overview

- Place injections in the lip line safety zone (Fig. 3).
  - **Upper lip safety zone** is at least 1 cm from the lateral corners of the mouth, 0.5 cm or less from the vermillion border, and extends to the lateral edge of the philtral column (Fig. 3A).
  - **Lower lip line safety zone** is at least 2 cm from the lateral corners of the mouth and is 0.5 cm or less from the vermillion border (Fig. 3B).
- An overview of injection points and OBTX doses for treatment of lip lines is shown in Figure 4. The upper lip requires one injection per side (Fig. 4A). The lower lip typically requires three injections, two laterally and one in the midline (Fig. 4B).

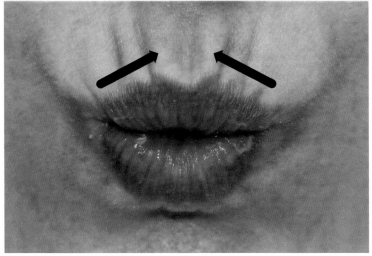

A   = 2.5 units Botox, insert needle in direction of arrow

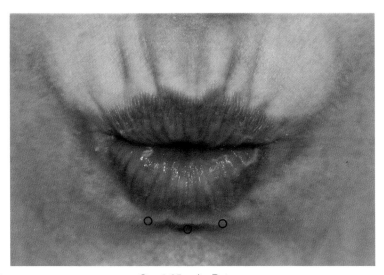

B   O = 1.25 units Botox

FIGURE 4 ● Overview of botulinum toxin injection points and doses in the upper **(A)** and lower **(B)** lips for treatment of lip lines. Copyright R. Small, MD.

- Marking injection points with the muscle contracted before anesthesia is helpful
  because once anesthetized, patients are unable to contract this muscle.
- Botulinum toxin is injected subdermally using a threading technique for treatment of
  upper lip lines. Superficial injection is important to avoid the deeper muscles, which
  insert in the lip area and affect lip function.
- Injecting too deep or lateral to the lip line safety zone may involve muscles that control
  lip function and increase the risk of oral incompetence.
- Injecting medial to the lip line safety zone, into the philtral columns, may result in
  an undesired flattening of the Cupid's bow.

- Take care to inject equal doses bilaterally to avoid lip asymmetry.
- In patients who have never had botulinum toxin treatment of the lips, and for providers who are getting started with lip line botulinum toxin treatments, it is advisable to treat only the upper or the lower lip in a given visit.

Technique

1. Position the patient at a 60-degree reclined position.
2. Identify the lip line safety zone (Fig. 3).
3. Locate the orbicularis oris muscle by instructing the patient to contract the muscle using one of the facial expressions above.
4. Identify the injection points (Fig. 4). With the orbicularis oris muscle contracted, mark the two injection points on the upper lip in the ridges of the muscle, near the vermillion border, at least 1 cm from the corners of the mouth.
5. Apply topical anesthetic to the treatment area for 10–15 minutes and remove before treatment.
6. Apply ice for anesthesia to the side of the upper lip to be treated.
7. Prepare injection sites with alcohol and allow to dry.
8. The provider is positioned on the side that is to be injected.
9. While the mouth is at rest, insert the needle into the first injection point and thread superficially, such that the needle tip ends at the lateral edge of the philtral column. Use the first finger of the noninjecting hand to gently palpate the needle tip in the tissue and confirm placement. Inject 2.5 units with gentle, even plunger pressure as the needle is withdrawn (Fig. 5).
10. Compress the injection sites firmly to relieve discomfort.

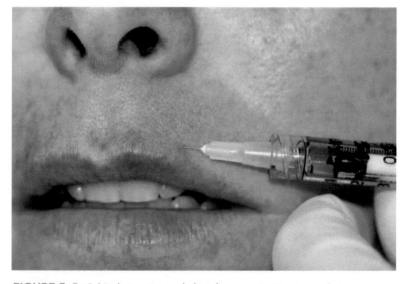

FIGURE 5 ● Orbicularis oris muscle botulinum toxin injection technique.
Copyright R. Small, MD.

11. Apply ice for anesthesia to the contralateral side of the upper lip to be treated.
12. Prepare injection sites with alcohol and allow to dry.
13. Repeat the above technique for the contralateral side of the upper lip.

Results

- **Reduction of dynamic lip lines** is typically seen 2 weeks after botulinum toxin treatment (see Figs. 1A and 1B).
- **Lip eversion with enhanced lip fullness** is also evident 2 weeks after botulinum toxin treatment (see Figs. 2A and 2B).
- **Preservation of the philtral columns** and **Cupid's bow,** with **minimal functional impairment of the mouth,** such that routine functions of eating, drinking, and speaking remain unaffected, are also desirable outcomes. Difficulty with puckering tightly, whistling, blowing a wind instrument, and sipping from a straw are anticipated and indicate that an adequate dose has been used.

Duration of Effects and Treatment Intervals

- Muscle function in the treatment area gradually returns by about 2 months after botulinum toxin treatment.
- Subsequent lip line treatments with botulinum toxin may be performed when function of the orbicularis oris muscle is regained and muscle ridges are visible.

Follow-Ups and Management

Patients are assessed 2 weeks after botulinum toxin treatment to evaluate for reduction of dynamic lip lines, lip eversion and preservation of oral function. Below are some commonly encountered follow-up issues:

- **Mild oral functional impairment.** Patients may complain of difficulty enunciating the letters "p" and "b," swishing and spitting after brushing teeth, or difficulty sipping from a spoon. These effects typically resolve spontaneously by 2 weeks. If they are bothersome to the patient or are prolonged for more than 2 weeks, decrease the OBTX dose in the upper lip to 1 unit per side at subsequent treatments.
- **Persistent lip lines.** If lip lines are present, evaluate for the following common causes:
  - **Orbicularis oris muscle contraction.** Patients may have greater muscle mass than anticipated in the treatment area and additional botulinum toxin may be required to achieve desired results. Excessive orbicularis oris muscle function can be reduced with a touch-up procedure using 1.25 units of OBTX per side, depending on the degree of muscle activity present. Botulinum toxin is injected in the areas with excessive contractility demonstrating muscle ridges. Reassess patients 2 weeks after the touch-up. The efficacious dose of botulinum toxin for treatment of the upper lip is determined to be the initial dose plus the touch-up dose. Start with this total dose at the patient's subsequent upper lip treatment in approximately 2–3 months.

- **Static lines**. If static lines are present, patients may require several consecutive botulinum toxin treatments for improvements to be seen. Combining botulinum toxin with other minimally invasive aesthetic procedures can offer enhanced results for treatment of static lip lines (see Combining Aesthetic Treatments below).

Complications and Management

- General injection-related complications (see Introduction and Foundation Concepts section, Complications)
- Lip asymmetry
- Alteration of lip shape (static or dynamic)
- Oral incompetence with resultant drooling, impaired speaking, eating, or drinking

    Lip asymmetry can result from unequal injection of botulinum toxin in the treatment area. This is rare and can be corrected by injecting small amounts of botulinum toxin into areas with excessive muscle contraction. The dose used will depend on the degree of muscle activity present, but typically 1.25 units of OBTX are placed in the areas of excessive contractility.

    Alteration of lip shape, particularly flattening of the Cupid's bow, can result from medial injection of botulinum toxin in the philtral columns. Lip shape will be restored as botulinum toxin effects diminish.

    Oral incompetence is a severe and rare complication, which can result in drooling, impaired speaking, eating, or drinking. Injecting too deeply or too laterally may involve the muscles that are important for oral competence. There is no corrective treatment for this complication and lip function will be regained as botulinum toxin effects diminish.

Botulinum Toxin Treatments in Multiple Areas

- **Upper and lower lips.** When getting started with botulinum toxin treatment of the lips, it is advisable to take a conservative approach and treat only the upper or the lower lip at the initial visit. Upper lip lines are a more common complaint than lower lip lines, and therefore, botulinum toxin treatment of the lips usually starts with the upper lip. After patients have successfully received at least one treatment of the upper lip with an efficacious botulinum toxin dose that achieves a favorable aesthetic effect with minimal to no compromise of oral functioning, patients may then receive treatment of the lower lip concomitantly with treatment of the upper lip.
- **Lower face.** The lower face is a highly functional region, responsible for speaking, eating, and drinking. It is therefore advisable to use a conservative approach to treatment in this region by rotating treatment areas, such that only one area is treated with botulinum toxin at any give time (see Introduction and Foundation Concepts section, Botulinum Toxin Treatments in Multiple Facial Areas).

Combining Aesthetic Treatments and Maximizing Results

- **Static lip lines.** Static lip lines respond well to a combination of botulinum toxin and dermal fillers and skin resurfacing procedures such as fractional ablative lasers.

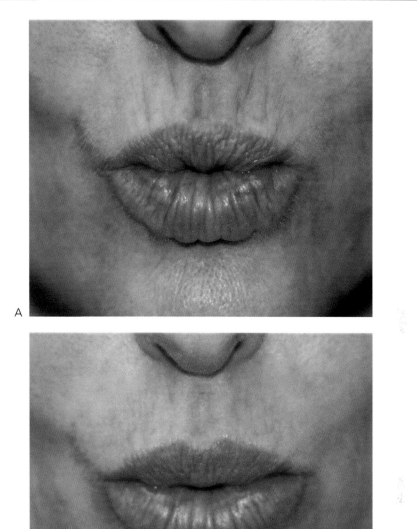

FIGURE 6 ● Upper lip lines before **(A)** and 1 month after **(B)** combination treatment with botulinum toxin and dermal filler above the upper lip, with active muscle contraction. Copyright R. Small, MD.

Figure 6 shows a patient before (Fig. 6A) and after (Fig. 6B) receiving a combination of botulinum toxin (Botox) and dermal filler (Radiesse® manufactured by Merz Aesthetics, Inc, San Mateo, CA) above the upper lip. Figure 7 shows a patient with more severe radial lip lines before (Fig. 7A) and after (Fig. 7B) receiving a combination of botulinum toxin (Botox), dermal filler (Radiesse), and fractional ablative skin resurfacing with an erbium laser (DermaSculpt manufactured by HOYA ConBio, Fremont, CA) above the upper lip.

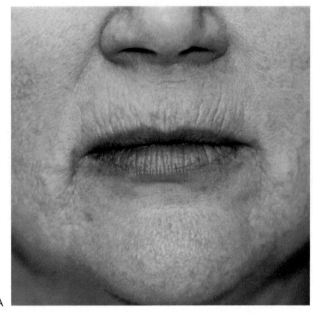

A

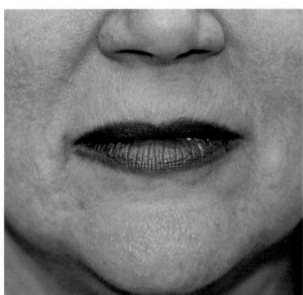

B

FIGURE 7 ● Upper lip lines before **(A)** and 1 month after **(B)** combination treatment with botulinum toxin, dermal filler, and fractional ablative laser resurfacing above the upper lip. Copyright R. Small, MD.

Pricing

Charges for botulinum toxin treatment of the upper lip or the lower lip range from $125–$200 per treatment or $25–$40 per unit of OBTX. This is an advanced treatment area and the unit price is greater than that for the basic areas of the upper face.

Chapter 8

Gummy Smile

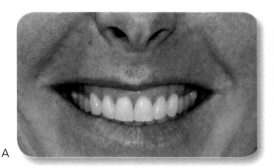
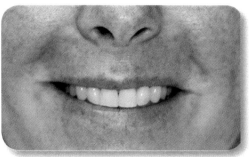

A

B

FIGURE 1 ● Gummy smile before **(A)** and 2 weeks after **(B)** botulinum toxin treatment of the levator labii superioris alaeque nasi muscle, while smiling. Copyright R. Small, MD.

Exaggerated upper lip retraction during smiling can result in a gummy smile with excessive gingival show. Gummy smiles associated with deep nasolabial folds result from contraction of the levator labii superioris alaeque nasi muscle. Treatment of the levator labii superioris alaeque nasi with botulinum toxin inhibits muscle contraction, which lengthens the upper lip reducing gingival show, and also reduces nasolabial folds.

Indications

- Gummy smile
- Nasolabial folds

Anatomy

- **Aesthetic norms.** A **gummy smile** reveals excessive gingiva, typically more than 2 mm above the central incisors, and is associated with inversion and thinning of the upper lip. The aesthetic norm for smiling is an upper lip covering the upper third of the central incisors during smiling.
- **Muscles targeted.** A gummy smile associated with a deep nasolabial fold results from contraction of the levator labii superioris alaeque nasi muscle (see Anatomy section,

Figs. 1 and 2) and is amenable to treatment with botulinum toxin as outlined in this chapter.

- **Muscle functions.** The levator labii superioris alaeque nasi muscle engages with smiling to function as a medial lip levator and contributes to formation of nasolabial folds (see Anatomy section, Fig. 7 and Table 1).
- **Muscles avoided.** A gummy smile associated with a flat nasolabial fold usually results from contraction of the levator labii superioris muscle, which is not amenable to botulinum toxin treatment. Other levator muscles that contribute to smile formation such as the levator anguli oris, zygomaticus major, and zygomaticus minor are also avoided with botulinum toxin treatment for a gummy smile (see Anatomy section, Fig. 3).

Patient Assessment

- **Social history** is obtained, including occupations/activities necessitating full oral competence, such as wind instrument musicians, actors, singers, and public speakers.
- **Gingival show with smiling** is assessed as follows:
  - **Gummy smiles associated with deep nasolabial folds** are amenable to botulinum toxin treatment using the technique outlined in this chapter.
  - **Gummy smiles and flat nasolabial folds** are not amenable to treatment with botulinum toxin.
- **Smile asymmetry** is assessed, and if present, pointed out to the patient before treatment.
- **Static lip structure** is assessed. The best candidates for treatment of a gummy smile often have upper lip retraction in which their upper incisors are visible at rest. The risk of excessive lip lengthening in these patients is minimal.

Eliciting Contraction of Muscles to Be Treated

Instruct the patient to perform the following expression:

- "Smile as hard as you can"

Treatment Goal

- Partial inhibition of the inferior labii superioris alaeque nasi muscle.

Reconstitution

- Reconstitute 100 units of Botox Cosmetic powder with 4 mL of nonpreserved saline (see Introduction and Foundation Concepts section, Reconstitution Method).
- Botulinum toxin products are not interchangeable and all references in this chapter to onabotulinumtoxinA (OBTX) refer specifically to Botox.

Starting Doses

- Women and men: total (bilateral) dose is 2.5 units of OBTX.

Anesthesia

- Anesthesia is not necessary for most patients but an ice pack may be used if required.

Equipment for Treatment

- General botulinum toxin injection supplies (see Introduction and Foundation Concepts section, Equipment)
- Reconstituted Botox Cosmetic
- 30-gauge, 0.5-inch needle

Procedure Overview

- An overview of injection points and OBTX doses for treatment of a gummy smile is shown in Figure 2.
- Treatment of a gummy smile requires precise injection into the levator labii superioris alaeque nasi muscle and the outcome is highly dependent on the botulinum toxin dose and injection location.
- Botulinum toxin is injected intramuscularly for treatment of a gummy smile and the levator labii superioris alaeque nasi must be clearly visible for treatment to be performed.
- Injecting laterally may involve other lip levator muscles and increase the risk of smile asymmetry and oral incompetence.

Technique

1. Position the patient at a 60-degree reclined position.
2. Locate the levator labii superioris alaeque nasi muscle by instructing the patient to contract the muscle using the facial expression above.
3. Identify the injection points (Fig. 2).
4. Ice for anesthesia (optional).
5. Prepare injection sites with alcohol and allow them to dry.

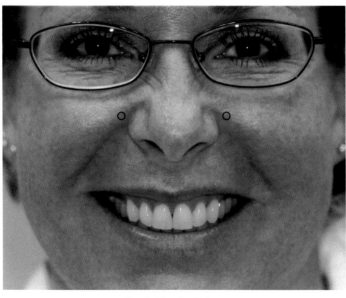

O = 1.25 units Botox

FIGURE 2 ● Overview of botulinum toxin injection points and doses for treatment of a gummy smile. Copyright R. Small, MD.

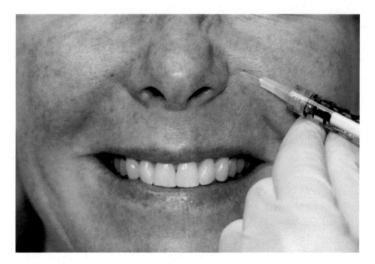

FIGURE 3 ● Levator labii superioris alaeque nasi muscle botulinum toxin injection technique. Copyright R. Small, MD.

6. The provider is positioned on the same side that is to be injected.
7. While the levator labii superioris alaeque nasi muscle is contracted, insert the needle in the muscle bulge at the uppermost part of the nasolabial fold (Fig. 3). The needle is angled medially and inserted to half the needle length. Inject 1.25 units of OBTX.
8. Compress the injection sites medially.
9. Repeat for the contralateral side of the face.

Results

- **Lengthening of the upper lip with reduction of gummy smile, and reduction of nasolabial folds** are evident 2 weeks after botulinum toxin treatment. Figure 1 shows a gummy smile and deep nasolabial fold with contraction of the levator labii superioris alaeque nasi muscle before (Fig. 1A) and 2 weeks after (Fig. 1B) botulinum toxin injection. Note that before treatment, the upper lip appears inverted and thinned whereas after treatment, lip fullness is enhanced.
- **Minimal or no functional impairment of the mouth** such that routine functions of eating, drinking, and speaking are unaffected, is also a desirable outcome.

Duration of Effects and Treatment Intervals

- Muscle function in the treatment area gradually returns by about 2 months after botulinum toxin injection.
- Subsequent treatments with botulinum toxin may be performed when function of the levator labii superioris alaeque nasi muscle is regained.

Follow-Ups and Management

Patients are assessed 2 weeks after botulinum toxin treatment to evaluate for reduction of a gummy smile with lengthening of the upper lip, reduction of nasolabial folds, oral function, and asymmetries. Some commonly encountered follow-up issues are as follows:

- **Persistent gummy smile.** It is desirable for patients to retain some levator labii superioris alaeque nasi muscle function, visible as elevation of the upper lip with smiling. However, if the treated labii superioris alaeque nasi muscle has excessive muscle strength after treatment and gingival show is not reduced relative to the pre-treatment appearance, additional botulinum toxin may be required to achieve desired results. A touch-up procedure may be performed with 1.25 units of OBTX using the same method described above. Reassess 2 weeks after the touch-up. The dose of botulinum toxin for treatment of the labii superioris alaeque nasi muscle is determined to be the initial dose plus the touch-up dose. Start with this total dose at the patient's subsequent gummy smile treatment in approximately 2 months.

Complications and Management

- General injection-related complications (see Introduction and Foundation Concepts section, Complications)
- Smile asymmetry
- Lip ptosis
- Other lip asymmetry or alteration of lip shape (static or dynamic)
- Oral incompetence with resultant drooling or impaired elocution, eating, or drinking

Complications can occur frequently with treatment of gummy smiles. Patients often have **asymmetric smiles** at baseline, which they may not be aware of. A subtle pretreatment lip asymmetry may become exaggerated after symmetric botulinum toxin treatment of the levator labii superioris alaeque nasi muscle. Lip asymmetry may also result from unequal botulinum toxin doses administered to the levator labii superioris alaeque nasi muscle. In either case, a smile asymmetry may be corrected with a touch-up procedure (as outlined above), with injection on the side that has greater muscle contractility.

Lip ptosis may result from complete relaxation of the levator labii superioris alaeque nasi muscle with excessive dosing of botulinum toxin. Lateral injection or diffusion of botulinum toxin into other lip levator muscles (levator labii superioris, levator anguli oris, zygomaticus major, and zygomaticus minor) can also result in lip ptosis and/or **impair oral competence** resulting in drooling, or impaired elocution, eating, or drinking. There is no corrective treatment for these complications and they improve spontaneously as botulinum toxin effects wear off over 2 months.

Botulinum Toxin Treatments in Multiple Lower Face Areas

The lower face is a highly functional region, responsible for speaking, eating, and drinking. It is, therefore, advisable to use a conservative approach to treatment in this region by rotating treatment areas, such that only one area is treated with botulinum toxin at any give time (see Introduction and Foundation Concepts section, Botulinum Toxin Treatments in Multiple Facial Areas).

Combining Aesthetic Treatments and Maximizing Results

- **Upper lip enhancement.** Patients who present with a gummy smile and deep nasolabial folds often have a thin upper lip as well. These patients can often benefit from combining botulinum toxin treatment of the levator labii superioris alaeque nasi muscle with dermal filler in the body of the lips. Dermal filler alone often yields suboptimal results in these patients.

- **Nasolabial folds.** Nasolabial folds respond well to dermal filler treatment alone and rarely require combination treatment with botulinum toxin in the levator labii superioris alaeque nasi muscle.

Pricing

Charges for botulinum toxin treatment of a gummy smile range from \$125–\$200 per treatment or \$25–\$40 per unit of OBTX. This is an advanced treatment area and the price per unit is greater than that for the basic areas of the upper face.

Chapter 9

Marionette Lines

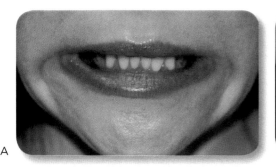
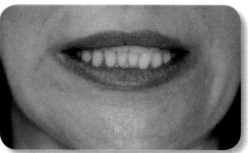

A
B

FIGURE 1 ● Marionette lines before **(A)** and 2 weeks after **(B)** botulinum toxin treatment of the depressor anguli oris muscle, with active muscle contraction. Copyright R. Small, MD.

Marionette lines and down-turned corners of the mouth result from contraction of the depressor anguli oris muscle as well as the loss of perioral soft-tissue density. These lines can give the face a sad or sullen expression. Treatment of the depressor anguli oris with botulinum toxin inhibits muscle contraction, resulting in elevation of the corners of the mouth and reduction of marionette lines.

Indications

- Marionette lines
- Elevation of down-turned corners of the mouth
- Enhanced smile

Anatomy

- **Wrinkles.** Marionette lines, or melomental folds, extend inferiorly from the oral commissures toward the jaw line (see Anatomy section, Figs. 4 and 5). The oral commissure is the junction between the upper and lower lip at the corner of the mouth.

97

- **Muscles targeted.** Botulinum toxin treatment of marionette lines targets the depressor anguli oris muscle. This triangular shaped muscle originates on the mandibular border and inserts on the corner of the mouth. The superior platysma muscle interdigitates with the depressor anguli oris near the mandible and can also contribute to marionette line formation (see Anatomy section, Figs. 1 and 2).
- **Muscle functions.** The depressor anguli oris muscle is activated with frowning and functions to draw the corners of the mouth inferiorly (see Anatomy section, Fig. 7 and Table 1). It antagonizes the levator muscles of the corners of the mouth (levator anguli oris, zygomaticus major, and zygomaticus minor), which are activated with smiling. Adequate strength of the depressor anguli oris is required for moving food intraorally with mastication and also functions to limit elevation of the corners of the mouth with smiling.
- **Muscles avoided.** The depressor labii inferioris muscle, a central lip depressor, lies medial to the depressor anguli oris muscle and is avoided with treatment of marionette lines. The buccinator muscle, involved in flattening the cheek, lies lateral to the depressor anguli oris and is also avoided (see Anatomy section, Fig. 3).

Patient Assessment

- **Social history** is obtained, including occupations/activities necessitating full oral competence such as wind instrument musicians, actors, singers, and public speakers.
- **Dynamic** (with muscle contraction) and **static** (at rest) **marionette lines** and **downturned corners of the mouth** are assessed.

Eliciting Contraction of Muscles to Be Treated

Instruct the patient to perform any of the following expressions:

- "Clench your teeth and pull the corners of your mouth downward"
- "Show me your bottom teeth"
- "Grimace"
- Say "ew" or "eek"

Treatment Goal

- Partial inhibition of the depressor anguli oris muscle.

Reconstitution

- Reconstitute 100 units of Botox Cosmetic powder with 4 mL of nonpreserved saline (see Introduction and Foundation Concepts section, Reconstitution Method).
- Botulinum toxin products are not interchangeable and all references in this chapter to onabotulinumtoxinA (OBTX) refer specifically to Botox.

Starting Doses

- Women and men: total (bilateral) dose is 5 units of OBTX.

Anesthesia

- Anesthesia is not necessary for most patients but an ice pack may be used if required.

Equipment for Treatment

- General botulinum toxin injection supplies (see Introduction and Foundation Concepts section, Equipment)
- Reconstituted Botox Cosmetic
- 30-gauge, 0.5-inch needle

Procedure Overview

- Place injections within the marionette line safety zone (Fig. 2). The safety zone is at least 1 cm anterior to the border of the masseter muscle, posterior to the marionette line, and within 2 cm of the mandibular margin. The anterior margin of the masseter muscle can be identified by palpating the middle of the mandible and directing the patient to contract the masseter muscle by clenching their teeth. The marionette line is a perpendicular line drawn from the corner of the mouth to the jaw at rest.

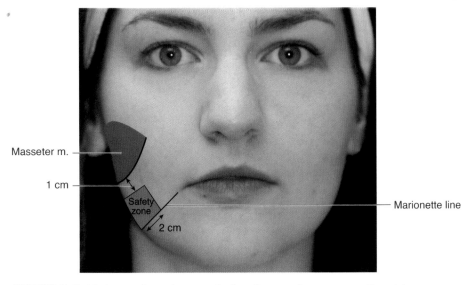

FIGURE 2 ● Marionette line safety zone for botulinum toxin treatments. Copyright R. Small, MD.

- An overview of injection points and OBTX doses for treatment of marionette lines is shown in Figure 4, from the front (Fig. 4A) and oblique (Fig. 4B) views. Treatment of marionette lines requires only one injection per side.
- Precise injection at the depressor anguli oris muscle is achieved through visualization and direct palpation of the contracted muscle. If the depressor anguli oris muscle cannot be identified, treatment of marionette lines with botulinum toxin should not be performed.
- Botulinum toxin is injected intramuscularly for treatment of marionette lines.
- Injecting inferior to the marionette line safety zone may involve muscles that control the central lower lip, such as the depressor labii inferioris, increasing the risk of lip asymmetry.
- Injecting lateral to the marionette line safety zone may involve the cheek buccinator muscle, increasing the risk of cheek flaccidity.
- Injecting too close to the lip outside of the marionette line safety zone may involve the orbicularis oris, increasing the risk or oral incompetence.

Technique

1. Position the patient at a 60-degree reclined position.
2. Identify the marionette line safety zone (Fig. 2).
3. Locate of the inferior portion of the depressor anguli oris muscle that lies within the safety zone by instructing the patient to contract the muscle, using one of the facial expressions above, and palpate the muscle (Fig. 3).
4. Identify the injection points. The needle insertion point is at the intersection of the lateral canthal line and the nasolabial fold line (Figs. 4A and 4B).

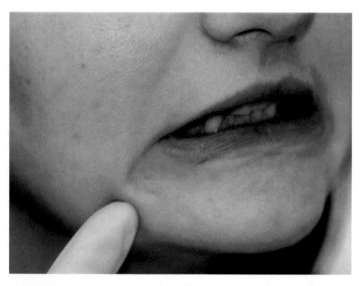

FIGURE 3 ● Depressor anguli oris muscle palpation. Copyright R. Small, MD.

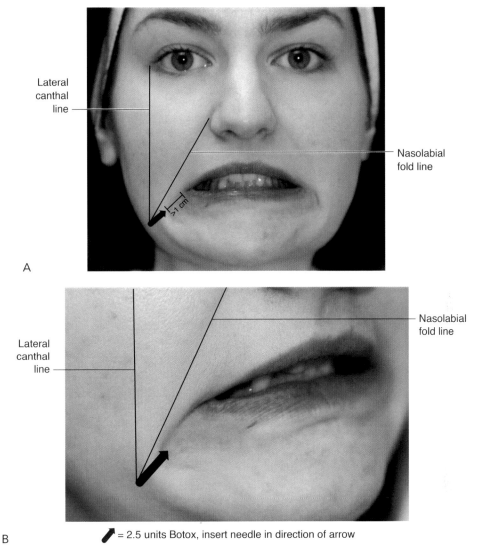

A

B

➤ = 2.5 units Botox, insert needle in direction of arrow

FIGURE 4 ● Overview of botulinum toxin injection points and doses for treatment of marionette lines: **(A)** front and **(B)** oblique view. Copyright R. Small, MD.

5. Ice for anesthesia (optional).
6. Prepare injection sites with alcohol and allow to dry.
7. The provider is positioned on the same side that is to be injected.
8. While the depressor anguli oris muscle is contracted, insert the needle in the depressor anguli oris muscle, at least 1 cm inferior to the corner of the lip. Angle the needle towards the corner of the mouth with the tip at the depressor anguli muscle. Inject 2.5 units of OBTX (Fig. 5).
9. Compress the injection sites firmly in an inferior direction.
10. Repeat this injection technique for the contralateral side of the face.

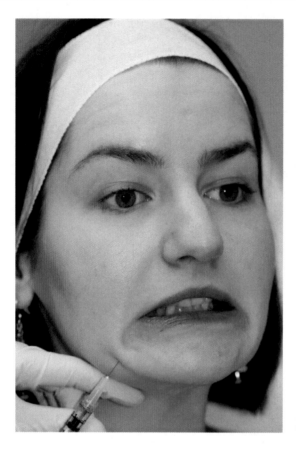

FIGURE 5 ● Depressor anguli oris
muscle botulinum toxin injection
technique. Copyright R. Small, MD.

Results

- **Reduction of dynamic marionette lines, depressor anguli oris muscle strength**
  and **elevation of the corners of the mouth** are evident 2 weeks after botulinum toxin treatment. Figure 1 shows contraction of the depressor anguli oris
  muscle before (Fig. 1A) and 2 weeks after (Fig. 1B) botulinum toxin injection.
  Botulinum toxin treatment results in the lower face are subtle, relative to the
  dramatic changes seen in the upper third of the face. Patients may appreciate
  pre- and posttreatment dynamic improvements if they are schooled in how to make
  these assessments with animation. However, they may not be able to appreciate a
  difference when the face is static.
- **Minimal or no functional impairment of the mouth,** such that routine
  functions of eating, drinking, and speaking are unaffected, is also a desirable
  outcome.

Duration of Effects and Treatment Intervals

- Muscle function in the treatment area gradually returns by about 2–3 months after
  botulinum toxin injection.
- Subsequent treatments with botulinum toxin may be performed when function of the
  depressor anguli oris muscle is regained.

Follow-Ups and Management

Patients are assessed 2 weeks after botulinum toxin treatment to evaluate for weakening of the depressor anguli oris muscle, reduction of marionette lines, elevation of the corners of the mouth and retention of oral function. Some commonly encountered follow-up issues are as follows:

- **Persistent depressor anguli oris muscle strength.** Patients may retain depressor anguli oris strength if they have greater muscle mass than anticipated or with improper placement of botulinum toxin at the time of treatment. Excessive depressor anguli oris strength can be reduced with a touch-up procedure using 1.25–2.5 units of OBTX per side, depending on the degree of muscle activity present. Reassess 2 weeks after the touch-up. The efficacious dose of botulinum toxin for treatment of the depressor anguli oris muscle is determined to be the initial dose plus the touch-up dose. Start with this total dose at the patient's subsequent marionette lines treatment in approximately 2–3 months.
- **Persistent marionette lines.** Static marionette lines with down-turned corners of the mouth typically require combination treatment with dermal fillers to achieve dramatic improvements (see Combining Aesthetic Treatments given later).
- **Mild oral functional impairment.** Difficulty with swishing liquids (e.g., after brushing teeth) and mild food trapping in the lower gingivobuccal groove are anticipated, which indicate that an adequate dose has been used. These effects typically resolve spontaneously by 2–4 weeks.

Complications and Management

- General injection-related complications (see Introduction and Foundation Concepts section, Complications).
- Lip asymmetry or alteration of lip shape (static or dynamic).
- Cheek flaccidity.
- Oral incompetence with resultant drooling or impaired elocution, eating, or drinking.

Lip asymmetry can result from unequal injection of botulinum toxin in the depressor anguli oris muscles. Lowering of the corner of the mouth with depressor anguli oris muscle contraction is evident on the untreated side (Fig. 6) because of retained depressor function of the depressor anguli oris. This can be corrected by injection of small botulinum toxin doses in the untreated side, as described earlier, for treatment of persistent depressor anguli oris muscle strength.

Lip asymmetry may also result from medial injection or diffusion of botulinum toxin into the depressor labii inferioris muscle. The depressor labii inferioris functions to lower the central lip, and relaxation of this muscle with botulinum toxin, therefore, results in elevation of the lip (see Chin chapter, Fig. 6), which is most noticeable with smiling. This effect typically resolves spontaneously over 2–4 weeks. It may be corrected with injection of 1.25 units of OBTX in the unaffected depressor labii inferioris muscle. However, watchful waiting for botulinum toxin effects to spontaneously resolve is recommended for management if lip asymmetry due to depressor labii inferioris muscle involvement is not too significant.

Cheek flaccidity may result from lateral injection or diffusion of botulinum toxin into the buccinator muscle. Patients may experience difficulty with mastication and be predisposed to biting the cheek.

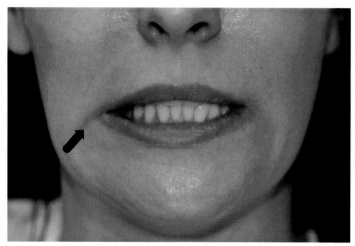

= 2.5 units Botox, insert needle in direction of arrow

FIGURE 6 ● Asymmetric depressor anguli oris muscle strength with increased contraction on the right side and correction with botulinum toxin. Copyright R. Small, MD.

Oral incompetence is a severe and rare complication that can result in drooling or impaired elocution, eating, or drinking. Injecting too close to the lip may involve the orbicularis oris muscle, which is important for oral competence. There is no corrective treatment for this complication and it improves spontaneously as the botulinum toxin effect wears off over 2–3 months.

Botulinum Toxin Treatments in Multiple Lower Face Areas

- The lower face is a highly functional region, responsible for speaking, eating, and drinking. It is, therefore, advisable to use a conservative approach to treatment in this region by rotating treatment areas, such that only one area is treated with botulinum toxin at any give time (see Introduction and Foundation Concepts section, Botulinum Toxin Treatments in Multiple Facial Areas).

Combining Aesthetic Treatments and Maximizing Results

- **Static marionette lines.** Static marionette lines and downturned oral commissures respond well to a combination of botulinum toxin and dermal fillers. Figure 7 shows a patient before (Fig. 7A) and after (Fig. 7B) receiving a combination of botulinum toxin (Botox) in the depressor anguli oris muscle and dermal filler (Juvederm; Allergan, Inc., Irvine, CA) in the marionette lines.

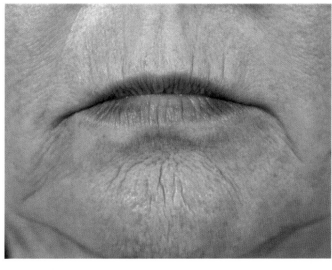

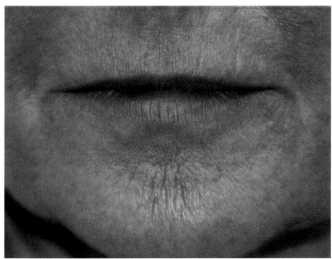

FIGURE 7 ● Marionette lines before **(A)** and after **(B)** combination treatment with botulinum toxin in the depressor anguli oris muscle and dermal filler in the marionette lines and oral commissures. Copyright R. Small, MD.

Pricing

Charges for botulinum toxin treatment of marionette lines range from $125–$200 per treatment or $25–$40 per unit of OBTX. This is an advanced treatment area and the price per unit is greater than that for the basic areas of the upper face.

Chapter 10

Chin

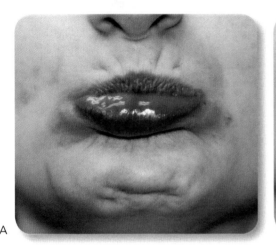 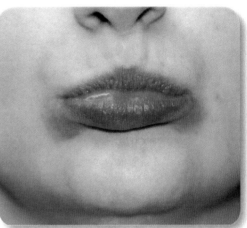

A   B

FIGURE 1 ● Puckered chin before **(A)** and 2 weeks after **(B)** botulinum toxin treatment of the mentalis muscle, with active pouting. Copyright R. Small, MD.

A puckered or cobblestoned appearance to the chin, and formation of a dynamic mental crease, result from contraction of the mentalis muscle. Treatment of the mentalis muscle with botulinum toxin inhibits contraction, which smoothes the chin surface and reduces the mental crease.

Indications

- Puckered or cobblestoned chin
- Mental crease

Anatomy

- **Wrinkles.** The mental crease, or labiomental crease, is a horizontal line inferior to the lower lip (see Anatomy section, Figs. 4 and 5). The mentalis muscle has numerous

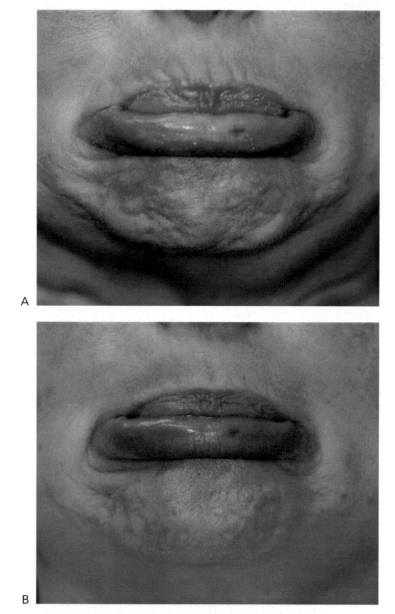

A

B

FIGURE 2 ● Pebbly chin before **(A)** and 2 weeks after **(B)** botulinum toxin treatment of the mentalis muscle, with active pouting. Copyright R. Small, MD.

attachments to the skin of the chin and contraction causes puckering and textural changes of the chin, referred to as a cobblestoned, pebbly, peach pit, dimpled, or *peau d'orange* appearance.

- **Muscles targeted.** Botulinum toxin chin treatment targets the mentalis muscle. This is a deep, two-bellied muscle. However, because of the superficial skin attachments, botulinum toxin is injected superficially (see Anatomy section, Figs. 1 and 2).
- **Muscle functions.** The mentalis muscle raises and protrudes the lower lip with pouting and drinking (see Anatomy section, Fig. 7 and Table 1).

- **Muscles avoided.** The depressor labii inferioris muscle, a central lip depressor, lies lateral to the mentalis muscle and is avoided with treatment of the chin. The orbicularis oris muscle lies superior to the mentalis muscle and is also avoided with treatment of the chin.

Patient Assessment

- **Social history** is obtained, including occupations/activities necessitating full oral competence, such as wind instrument musicians, actors, singers, and public speakers.
- **Dynamic puckering of the chin** and **mental crease formation** are assessed with contraction of the mentalis muscle. Patients are often unaware of chin puckering because it is most obvious during facial expressions when patients rarely observe themselves.
- **Static mental crease** is also assessed.

Eliciting Contraction of Muscles to Be Treated

Instruct the patient to perform following expression:

- "Pout"

Treatment Goal

- Partial inhibition of the mentalis muscle.

Reconstitution

- Reconstitute 100 units of Botox Cosmetic powder with 4 mL of nonpreserved sterile saline (see Introduction and Foundation Concepts, Reconstitution Method).
- Botulinum toxin products are not interchangeable and all references in this chapter to onabotulinumtoxinA (OBTX) refer specifically to Botox.

Starting Doses

- Women and men: total dose is 5 units of OBTX.

Anesthesia

- Anesthesia is not necessary for most patients but an ice pack may be used if required.

Equipment for Treatment

- General botulinum toxin injection supplies (see Introduction and Foundation Concepts section, Equipment)
- Reconstituted Botox Cosmetic
- 30-gauge, 0.5-inch needle

Procedure Overview

- Place injections within the chin safety zone (Fig. 3). The circumference of the chin is determined at rest, with the highest point at the mental crease. The safety zone is at least 1 cm medial to the chin circumference and is within 2 cm of the mandibular margin.

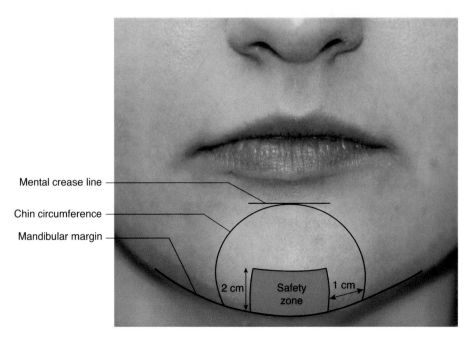

FIGURE 3 ● Chin safety zone for botulinum toxin treatments. Copyright R. Small, MD.

- Two techniques, based on the presenting chin shape, are commonly used for treating the chin. An overview of injection points and OBTX doses for these two methods is shown in Figure 4.
    - **Single injection technique,** with one medial injection point, is used for a narrow, rounded, or pointed chin (Fig. 4A).
    - **Double injection technique,** with one injection point on each side of the midline, is used for a broad, square, or cleft chin (Fig. 4B).
- Botulinum toxin is injected subdermally or superficial intramuscularly for treatment of chin puckering and the mental crease.
- Some patients engage several muscles, in addition to the mentalis muscle, with pouting, such as the depressor anguli oris and depressor labii inferioris, which can obscure the borders of the mentalis muscle and falsely give the appearance of a wide, square chin. If the mentalis muscle borders are indistinct, use the single injection technique to minimize the risk of injecting too laterally.
- Injecting lateral to the safety zone may involve the depressor labii inferioris muscle, resulting in lip asymmetry with elevation on the affected side.
- Injecting superior to the safety zone may involve the orbicularis oris muscle, resulting in functional impairment of the mouth.

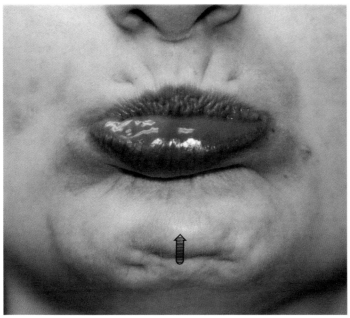

A   = 5 units Botox, insert needle in direction of arrow

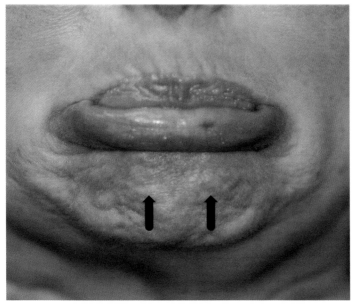

B   = 2.5 units Botox, insert needle in direction of arrow

FIGURE 4 ● Overview of botulinum toxin injection points and doses for treatment of the chin using single **(A)** and double **(B)** injection techniques. Copyright R. Small, MD.

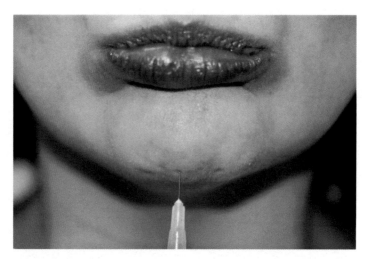

FIGURE 5 ● Botulinum toxin treatment of the mentalis muscle using the single injection technique. Copyright R. Small, MD.

Technique

1. Position the patient at a 60-degree reclined position.
2. Identify the chin safety zone (Fig. 3).
3. Locate the mentalis muscle by instructing the patient to contract the muscle using the facial expression above.
4. Select the single or double injection technique on the basis of the shape of the chin. Identify the injection points (Fig. 4).
5. Ice for anesthesia (optional).
6. Prepare injection sites with alcohol and allow to dry.
7. The provider is positioned in front of the patient.
8. **Single injection technique.** While the mentalis muscle is contracted, insert the needle just superior to the mandibular margin within the safety zone in the midline. Angle the needle and thread towards the lip such that the needle tip ends at the chin protuberance, at least 2 cm inferior to the vermillion border (Fig. 5). Inject 5 units of OBTX as the needle is slowly withdrawn, using gentle even plunger pressure.
9. **Double injection technique.** While the mentalis muscle is contracted, insert the needle lateral to the midline, just superior to the mandibular margin within the safety zone. Angle the needle and thread toward the lip such that the needle tip ends at the chin protuberance, at least 2 cm inferior to the vermillion border. Inject 2.5 units of OBTX in each site as the needle is slowly withdrawn, using gentle even plunger pressure. Repeat the above injection for the opposite site of the chin, equidistant from the midline.
10. Compress the injection sites firmly in an inferior direction.

Results

- **Smoothing of the chin** and **reduction of a dynamic mental crease** are evident 2 weeks after botulinum toxin treatment. Figure 1 shows contraction of the mentalis muscle in a patient with a narrow, rounded chin before (Fig. 1A) and 2 weeks after (Fig. 1B) botulinum toxin injection using the single injection technique. Figure 2 shows contraction of the mentalis muscle in a patient with a broader, square chin before (Fig. 2A) and 2 weeks after (Fig. 2B) botulinum toxin injection using the double injection technique. Note that this patient engages the depressor anguli oris muscle with pouting and, as anticipated, this muscle is still active after treatment of the mentalis muscle (Fig. 2B). Patients are able to appreciate pre- and posttreatment improvements when schooled in making dynamic assessments of the chin.

- **Minimal or no functional impairment of the mouth,** such that routine functions of eating, drinking, and speaking are unaffected, is also a desirable outcome.

Duration of Effects and Treatment Intervals

- Muscle function in the treatment area gradually returns by about 2–3 months after botulinum toxin injection.
- Subsequent treatments with botulinum toxin may be performed when function of the mentalis muscle is regained.

Follow-Ups and Management

Patients are assessed 2 weeks after botulinum toxin treatment to evaluate for weakening of the mentalis muscle and oral function. If persistent cobblestone or puckered appearance is present, evaluate for the following common causes:

- **Persistent chin puckering** and/or **dynamic mental crease.** It is desirable for patients to retain some mentalis muscle function, which may be visible as mild chin puckering or cobblestoning and mental crease formation. If significant puckering is present after treatment, with minimal chin smoothing relative to the pretreatment appearance, additional botulinum toxin may be required to achieve a desirable result. A touch-up procedure may be performed with 2.5 units or less of OBTX using the same method as described earlier. Reassess for aesthetic results and oral function 2 weeks after the touch-up. The efficacious dose of botulinum toxin for mentalis muscle treatment is determined to be the initial dose plus the touch-up dose. Start with this total dose at the patient's subsequent mentalis muscle treatment in approximately 2–3 months.
- **Static mental crease.** A static mental crease seen with the chin at rest, may improve with several consecutive botulinum toxin treatments. Combination treatment with dermal fillers is typically required to achieve a dramatic improvement.

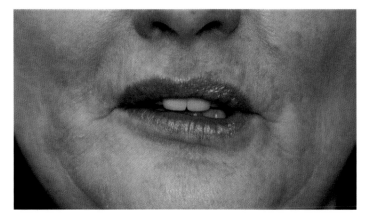

FIGURE 6 ● Lip asymmetry with elevation of the right lower lip due to weakening of the right depressor labii inferioris muscle with botulinum toxin. Copyright R. Small, MD.

Complications and Management

- General injection-related complications (see Introduction and Foundation Concepts section, Complications).
- Lip asymmetry or alteration of lip shape (static or dynamic).
- Oral incompetence with resultant drooling and impaired elocution, eating, or drinking.

Lip asymmetry or **alteration of lip shape** may result from lateral injection or diffusion of botulinum toxin into the depressor labii inferioris muscle. The depressor labii inferioris muscle functions to lower the central lip and relaxation of this muscle with botulinum toxin, therefore, results in elevation of the lip. Figure 6 shows lip asymmetry with elevation of the right lower lip due to weakening of the right depressor labii inferioris muscle with botulinum toxin. This effect typically resolves spontaneously over 2–4 weeks. Lower lip symmetry may be restored with injection of 1.25 units of OBTX into the unaffected depressor labii inferioris muscle. However, watchful waiting for botulinum toxin effects to spontaneously resolve is recommended for management if the lip asymmetry is not too bothersome to the patient.

Oral incompetence is a severe and rare complication, which can result in drooling or impaired elocution, eating, or drinking. Injecting too close to the lip may involve the orbicularis oris muscle, which is important for oral competence. Full immobilization of the mentalis muscle with excessively high botulinum toxin doses may also result in oral incompetence from impaired ability to elevate the lower lip. There are no corrective treatments for these complications and they improve spontaneously as the botulinum toxin effect wears off over 2–3 months.

Botulinum Toxin Treatments in Multiple Lower Face Areas

- The lower face is a highly functional region, responsible for speaking, eating, and drinking. It is, therefore, advisable to use a conservative approach to treatment in this region by rotating treatment areas, such that only one area is treated with botulinum toxin at any given time (see Introduction and Foundation Concepts section, Botulinum Toxin Treatments in Multiple Facial Areas).

Combining Aesthetic Treatments and Maximizing Results

- **Static mental crease.** Static mental creases respond well to combination treatment of botulinum toxin injection in the mentalis muscle and dermal fillers in the mental crease.

Pricing

Charges for botulinum toxin treatment of the mental crease range from $125–$250 per treatment or $25–$50 per unit of OBTX. This is an advanced treatment area and the price per unit is greater than that for the basic areas of the upper face.

Chapter 11

Neck Bands

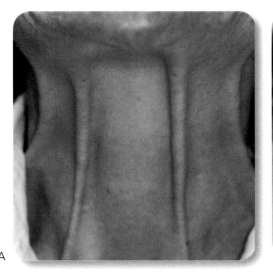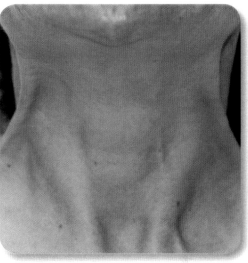

A   B

FIGURE 1 ● Neck bands before **(A)** and 2 weeks after **(B)** botulinum toxin treatment of the platysma muscle, with active muscle contraction. Copyright R. Small, MD.

Vertical neck bands result from contraction of the platysma muscle. Treatment of the platysma muscle with botulinum toxin inhibits contraction, which reduces neck band formation and submental fullness, resulting in a more defined neck contour.

Indications

- Neck bands
- Reduction of submental fullness, also referred to as neck lifting

Anatomy

- **Neck bands.** Neck bands, or platysmal bands, are typically two or more vertical folds that extend from the margin of the mandible to the clavicles (Fig. 1A). They are most

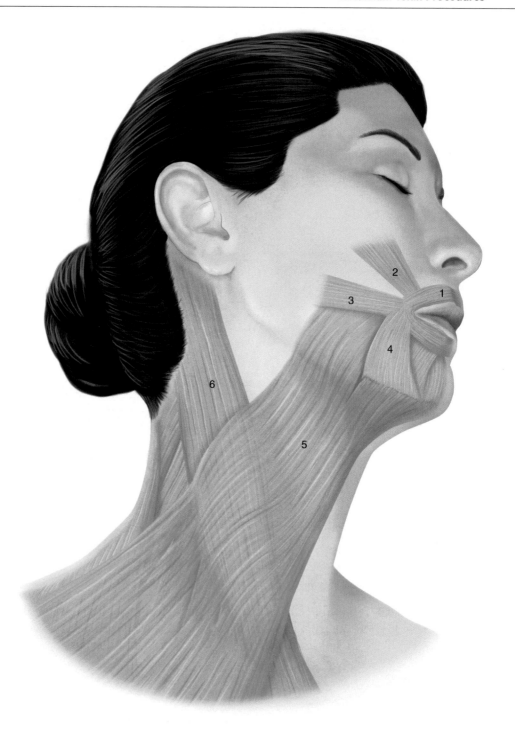

1. Orbicularis oris m.   4. Depressor anguli oris m.
2. Zygomaticus major m.   5. Platysma m.
3. Risorius m.   6. Sternocleidomastoid m.

FIGURE 2 ● Neck and lower face muscles. Copyright R. Small, MD.

evident with straining, for example when lifting a heavy weight or when speaking animatedly. Increased resting tone in the platysma muscle with age also contributes to platysmal band formation.

- **Muscle targeted.** Botulinum toxin neck band treatment targets the anterior neck platysma muscle. The platysma is a broad muscle that covers the anterior and lateral neck and the lower face (Fig. 2). It originates at pectoralis and deltoid muscles, extends over the clavicle, and inserts into different regions of the lower face.
- **Muscle functions.** The platysma muscle depresses the jaw and the corners of the mouth, expands the diameter of the neck, and in some cases, depresses the cheek. The anterior lower face fibers, which insert on the mandible, function as jaw depressors. The posterior lower face fibers, which pass over the mandible and interdigitate with the inferior perioral muscles such as the depressor anguli oris muscle, draw the corners of the mouth, and in some cases, the cheek, downward and laterally. The neck fibers expand the diameter of the neck.
- **Muscles avoided.** The platysma muscle overlies deeper neck muscles, including the sternocleidomastoid and laryngeal muscles, and is separated from them by a thin fascial layer. These deeper neck muscles are avoided with botulinum toxin treatment of neck bands.

Patient Assessment

- **Neck aging changes** are assessed, including platysmal bands, wrinkles, skin laxity, and increased adiposity.
  - **Platysmal muscle bands** are identified with platysma contraction while the patient is straining. These bands are responsive to treatment with botulinum toxin.
  - **Skin laxity and adiposity** are visible at rest. They are not improved with botulinum toxin treatment, and skin laxity may actually worsen with treatment. Figure 3 shows a patient at rest with lax skin folds that lie in a similar position to folds seen with platysmal neck bands. Lax skin folds and submental adiposity are not an indication for botulinum toxin treatment.
  - **Wrinkles** on the neck usually appear as static horizontal "necklace" lines. Some evidence suggests that horizontal neck lines improve with botulinum toxin treatments of the platysma muscle using a different method from that used to treat neck bands (see Other Neck Botulinum Toxin Treatments below).

Eliciting Contraction of Muscles to Be Treated

Instruct the patient to perform any of the following expressions:

- "Strain as if lifting heavy dumbbells with your arms"
- "Clench your teeth and pull the corners of your mouth downward"
- Say "ew" or "eek"

Treatment Goal

- Complete inhibition of the anterior neck platysma muscle.

Reconstitution

- Reconstitute 100 units of Botox Cosmetic powder with 4 mL of nonpreserved sterile saline (see Introduction and Foundation Concepts section, Reconstitution Method).

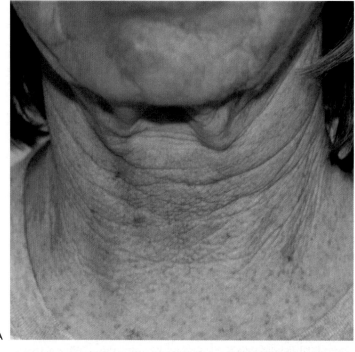
A

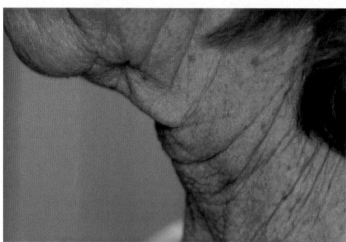
B

FIGURE 3 ● Skin laxity seen from the front **(A)** and lateral **(B)** views is not an indication for botulinum toxin treatment of the neck. Copyright R. Small, MD.

- Botulinum toxin products are not interchangeable and all references in this chapter to onabotulinumtoxinA (OBTX) refer specifically to Botox.

Starting Doses

- Women and men: 7.5–12.5 units of OBTX per neck band for a total of 15–25 units for two neck bands.

Anesthesia

- Anesthesia is not necessary for most patients but an ice pack may be used if required.

Equipment for Treatment

- General botulinum toxin injection supplies (see Introduction and Foundation Concepts section, Equipment)
- Reconstituted Botox Cosmetic
- 30-gauge, 0.5-inch needle

Procedure Overview

- Place injections within the neck band safety zone (Fig. 4). The safety zone is 1 cm lateral to the trachea and extends to the oral commissure lines, which are vertical lines extending inferiorly from the oral commissures to the clavicles. The safety zone is at least 2 cm inferior to the mandible and at least 4 cm superior to the clavicle margins.
- An overview of injection points and OBTX doses for treatment of neck bands is shown in Figure 5.
- Botulinum toxin is injected intramuscularly for treatment of neck bands. Intramuscular injection is achieved by grasping the neck band firmly between the first finger and

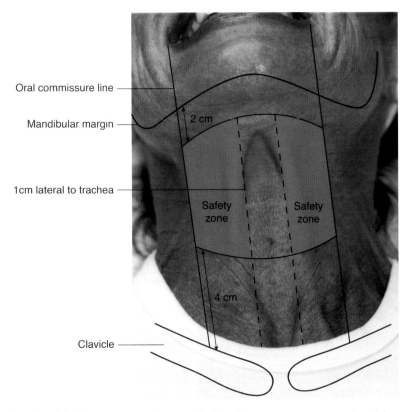

FIGURE 4 ● Neck band safety zone for botulinum toxin treatments. Copyright R. Small, MD.

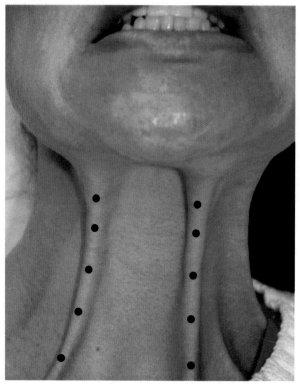

●= 2.5 units Botox

FIGURE 5 ● Overview of
botulinum toxin injection points
and doses for treatment of neck
bands. Copyright R. Small, MD.

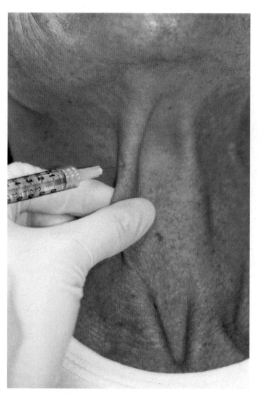

FIGURE 6 ● Platysma muscle botulinum
toxin injection technique. Copyright
R. Small, MD.

thumb using the nondominant hand (Fig. 6). The muscle ridge is palpable beneath the skin. The needle is angled medially, at about 45-degrees to the neck, and inserted into the band. A slight increase in resistance can be felt as the needle moves from skin into muscle. The tip of the 30-gauge 0.5-inch needle should just pass into the muscle ridge, and botulinum toxin injected at that site.

- When getting started with this procedure, it is advisable to treat neck bands located more medially in the safety zone and limit the treatment to no more than two neck bands.
- Injecting deeply may penetrate the neck fascia resulting in undesired spread of botulinum toxin to deeper neck muscles that are integral in deglutination and neck stability.
- Injecting medial to the safety zone in the midline may involve the laryngeal muscles affecting speech.

Technique

1. Position the patient at a 60-degree reclined position.
2. Identify the neck band safety zone (Fig. 4).
3. Locate the medial neck bands for treatment within the safety zone by instructing the patient to contract the muscles as directed above.
4. Identify the injection points (Fig. 5).
5. Ice for anesthesia (optional).
6. Prepare injection sites with alcohol and allow to dry.
7. The provider is positioned on the side that is to be injected.
8. While the platysma muscle is contracted, insert the needle at least 2 cm inferior to the jaw in the superior portion of the neck band. Direct the needle medially and ensure that the needle tip is intramuscular and not just in the skin, using the technique described in Overview above. Inject 2.5 units of OBTX (Fig. 6).
9. The next injection point is 1–2 cm inferior to the first and OBTX is injected using the same technique. Injections are continued inferiorly to the lower neck, with a total of 3–5 injection points per band, depending on the band length.
10. For the second neck band, repeat the injection technique above.
11. Compression is not typically required.

Results

- **Reduction of neck bands** is evident 2 weeks after botulinum toxin treatment. Figure 1 shows contraction of the platysma muscle before (Fig. 1A) and 2 weeks after (Fig. 1B) botulinum toxin injection.
- **Improved neck contour with reduction of submental fullness** at rest may also be evident 2 weeks after botulinum toxin treatment.

Duration of Effects and Treatment Intervals

- Muscle function in the treatment area gradually returns by about 3–5 months after botulinum toxin treatment.
- Subsequent treatments with botulinum toxin may be performed when function of the platysma muscle is regained.

Follow-Ups and Management

Patients are assessed 2 weeks after botulinum toxin treatment to evaluate for reduction of neck bands. Below is a commonly encountered follow-up issue:

- **Persistent neck bands with platysma muscle contraction.** Patients may have greater muscle mass than anticipated in the treatment area and additional botulinum toxin may be required to achieve desired results. A touch-up procedure may be performed with 2.5 units of OBTX per injection site in the active neck bands, using the same method as described above. The combined total dose for the initial treatment and touch-up procedure should not exceed 20 units of OBTX per neck band. Reassess 2 weeks after touch-up. The efficacious dose of botulinum toxin for treatment of the platysma muscle is determined to be the initial dose plus the touch-up dose. Start with this total dose at the patient's subsequent platysma muscle treatment in 3–5 months.

Complications and Management

- General injection-related complications (see Introduction and Foundation Concepts section, Complications)
- Dysarthria (difficulty articulating)
- Dysphagia (difficulty swallowing), and in severe cases nasogastric tube placement
- Hoarseness
- Neck weakness

Complications are rare with treatment of neck bands, however, when they occur, they can be significant and problematic.

Dysarthria may result from impaired oral function due to injection of botulinum toxin into the platysma muscle. The superior platysma muscle inserts on the muscles of the lower face and can affect function of the corners of the mouth, lower lip, and chin. Botulinum toxin injection in the superior portion of the platysma muscle, close to the mandibular margin, can, therefore, impair oral function.

Dysphagia neck weakness and **hoarseness** may result from spread of botulinum toxin to the deeper muscles that lie below the platysma muscle (such as the sternocleidomastoid and other strap muscles and laryngeal muscles of the neck). Dysphagia can occur with very high OBTX doses (≥180 units); however, there has been a case report of dysphagia requiring a nasogastric feeding tube with 60 units of OBTX injected in the neck. Neck weakness is typically reported as reduced neck flexion in the supine position. Hoarseness is due to diffusion of botulinum toxin to the laryngeal muscles. There are no corrective treatment for these complications and they improve spontaneously as botulinum toxin effects wears off over 3–4 months.

Other Neck Botulinum Toxin Treatments

Horizontal neck lines. Static horizontal neck lines, also called necklace lines, may be treated using 1–2 units of OBTX just above or below the line, within the neck band safety zone. Injections are intradermal, spaced 1.5–2 cm along the line. The most prominent horizontal line is the focus of treatment. It is advisable to avoid treating both neck bands and horizontal neck lines in the same visit, to limit botulinum toxin dosing in the neck.

Pricing

Charges for botulinum toxin treatment of neck bands range from $600–$800 per treatment for two neck bands or $25–$40 per unit of OBTX. This is an advanced treatment area and the price per unit is greater than that for the basic areas of the upper face.

Chapter 12

Axillary Hyperhidrosis

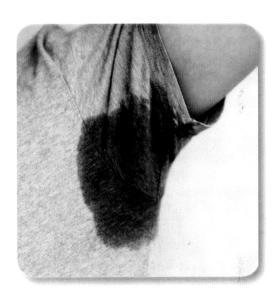

FIGURE 1 ● Axillary hyperhidrosis. Copyright R. Small, MD.

Primary axillary hyperhidrosis, defined as idiopathic focal excessive sweating, is estimated to affect more than 7.8 million people in the United States, with the highest incidence in adults aged 18–54 years. This condition impacts sufferers' quality of life through interference with social and occupational interactions and daily activities. Treatment of sweat glands in the dermis with botulinum toxin inhibits acetylcholine release, which decreases sweat production and reduces hyperhidrosis.

Indications

- Primary axillary hyperhidrosis

Anatomy

- **Sweat glands.** Sweat glands are located in the dermis and are sympathetically innervated by the acetylcholine neurotransmitter, which stimulates perspiration. Patients with axillary hyperhidrosis do not have an increased density of axillary sweat glands and the pathophysiologic mechanism of primary axillary hyperhidrosis is presumed to be due to sympathetic nervous system hyperactivity or dysregulation, resulting in excessive perspiration.

Patient Assessment

- **Diagnosis of primary axillary hyperhidrosis** is made after secondary causes of excessive sweating are excluded, such as spinal cord injury, peripheral nervous system pathology, hyperthyroidism, diabetes, malignancies, and others.
- **Diagnostic criteria** for primary axillary hyperhidrosis include focal, visible, and excessive sweating (Fig. 1) without apparent cause for at least 6 months' duration and at least two of the following:
  - Bilateral sweating.
  - Impairment in daily activities.
  - Frequency of at least one episode per week.
  - Age of onset less than 25 years.
  - Positive family history (65% of patients have a positive family history).
  - Cessation of focal sweating during sleep.
- **Hyperhidrosis Disease Severity Scale** is a self-reported qualitative tool that may be used to assess the severity of axillary hyperhidrosis. The degree of disruption to daily activities is categorized on a four-point scale, where a score of 3 or 4 is considered as severe hyperhidrosis.

  The Hyperhidrosis Disease Severity Scale is summarized in the table below.

Hyperhidrosis Disease Severity Scale	Description Underarm sweating is characterized as follows:
1	Never noticeable and never interferes with my daily activities.
2	Tolerable but sometimes interferes with my daily activities.
3	Barely tolerable and frequently interferes with my daily activities.
4	Intolerable and always interferes with my daily activities.

- A **stepwise treatment algorithm** is commonly used for axillary hyperhidrosis, which includes:
  - Initial therapy with over-the-counter antiperspirants.
  - Aluminum chloride 10–25% topical antiperspirant.
  - Intradermal injections of botulinum toxin.
  - Surgery with local sweat gland resection or endoscopic thoracic sympathectomy.

Treatment Goal

- Complete cessation of axillary perspiration or reduction of severity, such that the symptoms can be managed with over-the-counter antiperspirants.

Reconstitution

- Reconstitute 100 units of Botox Cosmetic powder with 4 mL of nonpreserved sterile saline (see Introduction and Foundation Concepts section, Reconstitution Method).
- Botulinum toxin products are not interchangeable and all references in this chapter to onabotulinumtoxinA (OBTX) refer specifically to Botox.

Starting Doses

- Women and men: 45–50 units of OBTX per axilla. A total of 20 injections per axilla are performed using 2.5 units of OBTX per injection point

Anesthesia

- Anesthesia is not necessary or most patients but an ice pack may be used if required.

Equipment for Iodine-Starch Test

- Iodine solution or swab (1–5%)
- Cornstarch
- Brush or gauze to wipe off excess starch
- Surgical marker
- Tape measure
- Alcohol
- Small sieve (optional)

Equipment for Treatment

- General botulinum toxin injection supplies (see Introduction and Foundation Concepts section, Equipment)
- Reconstituted Botox Cosmetic
- 30-gauge, 0.5-inch needle

Procedure Preparation and Overview

- Before treatment with botulinum toxin, the hyperhidrotic area is determined using the Minor's Iodine-Starch Test. Excessive perspiration is indicated with this test by a purple color change in the affected area when starch, iodine, and perspiration combine.
- To prepare for the starch-iodine test, patients are instructed to shave underarms and abstain from the use of over-the-counter deodorants or antiperspirants for 24 hours before the test.

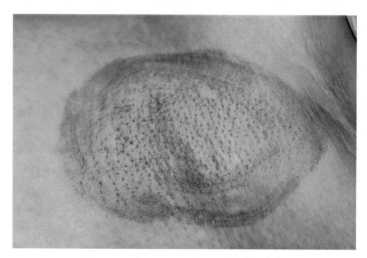

FIGURE 2 ● Axilla painted with iodine solution for iodine-starch test.
Copyright R. Small, MD.

- Botulinum toxin is injected intradermally for treatment of axillary hyperhidrosis. Effects may be diminished with deeper injection.
- Do not inject directly into ink marks to avoid inadvertently tattooing the skin.

Technique

Minor's Iodine-Starch Test

1. Position the patient supine on the treatment bed, with arms raised.
2. Dry the axilla and then paint with iodine solution, making sure to cover the area surrounding the axilla. Allow the iodine to dry (Fig. 2).
3. Sprinkle starch on the area using a sieve (Fig. 3).
4. Brush off excess starch powder and wait for 10 minutes (Fig. 4).
5. An intense purple color will be evident in the hyperhidrotic areas. Encircle the purple area with a surgical marker (Fig. 5) and document with photographs.
6. Clean the area inside the circle with alcohol to remove all the purple color and prepare the skin for injections. Use a surgical marker and tape measure to mark 20 evenly distributed injection points, 1.5–2 cm apart, per axilla (Fig. 6).

Botulinum Toxin Treatment

1. Using a 30-gauge 0.5-inch needle, inject 2.5 units of OBTX intradermally at each marked injection point. The needle is angled at 45-degrees to the skin surface, with the bevel up and the tip inserted just under the skin to approximately 2 mm in depth, to raise a wheal (Fig. 7). After injections, clean the area with alcohol to remove all marks.
2. Repeat this injection technique for the other axilla.
3. Compress injection sites.

Results

- Significant or complete reduction of underarm sweating occurs 1–2 weeks after treatment.

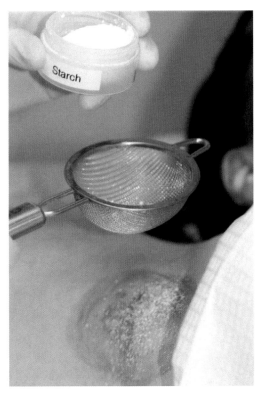

FIGURE 3 ● Starch powder applied to axilla for
iodine-starch test. Copyright R. Small, MD.

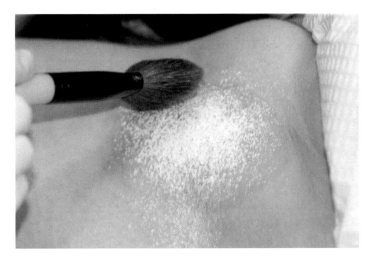

FIGURE 4 ● Excess starch powder removed for iodine-starch test.
Copyright R. Small, MD.

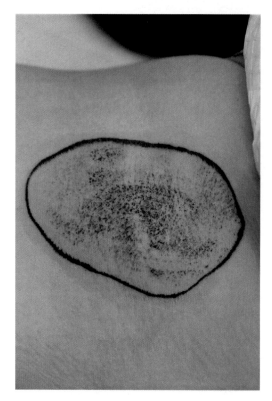

FIGURE 5 ● Circled hyperhidrotic area of purple coloration for iodine-starch test. Copyright R. Small, MD.

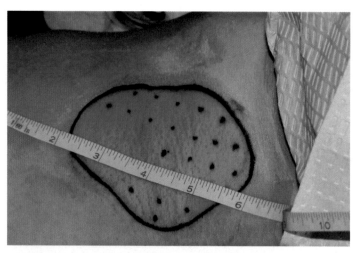

FIGURE 6 ● Injection points marked for botulinum toxin treatment of axillary hyperhidrosis. Copyright R. Small, MD.

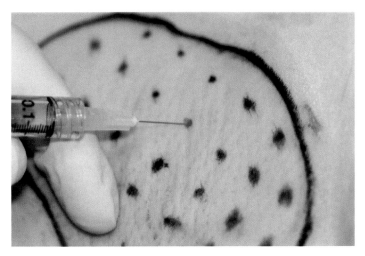

FIGURE 7 ● Intradermal injection technique for botulinum toxin treatment of axillary hyperhidrosis. Copyright R. Small, MD.

Duration of Effects and Treatment Intervals

• Perspiration gradually returns by about 6 months after botulinum toxin treatment and subsequent treatments with botulinum toxin may be performed at that time.

Follow-Ups and Management

Patients are assessed 2 weeks after botulinum toxin treatment to evaluate for reduction of perspiration. Follow-up issues are rare and include the following:

• **Persistent perspiration in the treatment area.** This can be corrected with a touch-up procedure using 2.5 units of OBTX per injection site in the area of residual perspiration. Patients may be able to identify the area where residual perspiration is occurring and the treatment directed there. Otherwise, an iodine-starch test may be performed to identify the areas of perspiration for the touch-up procedure. Touch-up procedures for axillary hyperhidrosis typically require 10–20 units of OBTX per axilla. At subsequent visits, use 45–50 units of OBTX, as it still may be possible to achieve an adequate response with this dose.

Complications and Management

• General injection-related complications (see Introduction and Foundation Concepts section, Complications)

Botulinum Toxin Treatments in Multiple Areas

• As the dose used for treatment of axillary hyperhidrosis is large, it is recommended that treatment of other areas with botulinum toxin be reserved for a separate visit.

Pricing

Charges for botulinum toxin treatment of bilateral axillary hyperhidrosis are typically $900–$1200 per treatment or $10–$12 per unit of OBTX.

Botulinum Toxin Treatment Tables

Botulinum Toxin Unit-to-Volume Conversion Table for Treatments

Botulinum Toxin Dose (units)	Botulinum Toxin Injection Volume (mL) Using a Reconstitution Concentration of 100 units/4 mL
1.25	0.05
2.50	0.10
3.75	0.15
5	0.20
7.5	0.30
10	0.40
12.5	0.50
15	0.60
17.5	0.70
20	0.80
22.5	0.90
25	1.00
27.5	1.10
30	1.20
32.5	1.30
35	1.40
37.5	1.50
40	1.60
42.5	1.70
45	1.80
47.5	1.90
50	2.00

APPENDIX 1. TABLE 2A

OnabotulinumtoxinA (Botox®) Starting Doses for Treatments

Treatment Areas	Muscles Targeted	Total[a] OBTX Dose (units)
Frown lines	Glabellar complex	20
Horizontal forehead lines	Frontalis	15
Crow's feet	Lateral orbicularis oculi	15
Lower eyelid wrinkles	Inferior preseptal orbicularis oculi	2.5
Eyebrow lift	Superior lateral orbicularis oculi	5
Bunny lines	Nasalis	2.5
Lip lines (upper)	Orbicularis oris	3.75
Gummy smile	Levator labii superioris alaeque nasi	2.5
Marionette lines	Depressor anguli oris	5
Chin	Mentalis	5
Neck bands	Platysma	15
Axillary hyperhidrosis	(Sweat glands)	45

[a]For treatment areas involving bilateral injection, this is the combined dose for both sides.
OBTX onabotulinumtoxinA (Botox)

APPENDIX 1. TABLE 2B

AbobotulinumtoxinA (Dysport®) Starting Doses for Treatments

Treatment Areas	Muscles Targeted	Total[a] ABTX Dose (units)
Frown lines	Glabellar complex	50
Horizontal forehead lines	Frontalis	30
Crow's feet	Lateral orbicularis oculi	30
Lower eyelid wrinkles	Inferior preseptal orbicularis oculi	4
Eyebrow lift	Superior lateral orbicularis oculi	12
Bunny lines	Nasalis	6
Lip lines (upper)	Orbicularis oris	8
Gummy smile	Levator labii superioris alaeque nasi	6
Marionette lines	Depressor anguli oris	10
Chin	Mentalis	10
Neck bands	Platysma	40
Axillary hyperhidrosis	(Sweat glands)	100

[a]For treatment areas involving bilateral injection, this is the combined dose for both sides.
ABTX abobotulinumtoxinA (Dysport)

Aesthetic Intake Form

Date:_____

NAME: _____ AGE:_____ * Date of Birth:_____

      Last,   First

ADDRESS: _____ CITY:_____ ZIP: _____

MOBILE PHONE: _____ ☐ OK TO CONTACT   ☐ LEAVE MESSAGE HERE

HOME PHONE: _____ ☐ OK TO CONTACT   ☐ LEAVE MESSAGE HERE

WORK PHONE: _____ ☐ OK TO CONTACT   ☐ LEAVE MESSAGE HERE

E-MAIL: _____ ☐ OK TO CONTACT

OCCUPATION: _____ How did you hear about us?: _____

In order of importance, beginning with 1, please rank what you would like to see improved in your skin:
_____ Reduction of wrinkles and fine lines _____ Reduction of brown spots/sun damage _____ Reduction of oil/acne _____ Reduction of Hair _____ Reduction of redness _____ Tattoo Removal _____ Other: _____
_____

Medical History	Yes	No	Please check all medical conditions past or present	Yes	No
Are you or is it possible that you may be pregnant?			Keloid scarring		
Are you breastfeeding?			Cold sores		
Do you form thick or raised scars from cuts or burns?			Herpes (genital)		

After injury to the skin (such as cuts/burns) do you have:
    Darkening of the skin in that area (hyperpigmentation)
    Lightening of the skin in that area (hypopigmentation)
			Easy bruising or bleeding		

			Active skin infection		
Hair removal by plucking, waxing, electrolysis or depilatory creams in the last 4 weeks?			Moles that have recently changed, itched, or bled		
Tanning (tanning bed) or sun expose in the last 4 weeks?			Recent increase in amount of hair		
Tanning products or spray on tan in the last 2 weeks?			Asthma		
Do you have a tan now in the area to be treated?			Seasonal allergies/ allergic rhinitis		

(Continued)

Medical History	Yes	No	Please check all medical conditions past or present	Yes	No
Do you use sunscreen daily with SPF 30 or higher?			Eczema		
Have you ever had a skin cancer? Type:			Thyroid imbalance		
List your common outdoor activities:			Poor healing		
Have you ever had a photosensitive disorder? (e.g. Lupus)			Diabetes		
Do you have a personal history of seizures?			Heart condition		
Permanent make-up or tattoos? Where:			High blood pressure		
Have you used Accutane in the last 6 months?			Pacemaker		
Are you currently taking any antibiotics? Which:			Disease of nerves or muscles (e.g. ALS, Myasthenia gravis, Lambert-Eaton or other)		
Are you using Retin-A or Glycolic products?			Cancer		
What is the name of your regular physician:			HIV/AIDS		
Do you have an allergy or sensitivity to lidocaine, latex, sulfa medications, hydroquinone, aloe, bee stings? (circle)			Autoimmune disease (e.g. rheumatoid arthritis, Scleroderma)		
Life threatening allergy to anything?			Hepatitis		
Do you currently smoke?			Shingles		
Do you have scars on the face?			Migraine headaches		
Explanation of items marked "Yes":			Other illness, health problems or medical conditions not listed:		

* For minors, please request Guardian information form.

I certify that the information I have given is complete and accurate.   _____Initials _____ Staff initials

For Internal Use Only Below This Line

_____

_____

_____

_____

Patient Information Handouts

3A. Botulinum Toxin Cosmetic Treatments

Before Treatment
- Avoid aspirin (e.g., Excedrin), vitamin E, St. John's wort, and other dietary supplements including ginkgo, evening primrose oil, garlic, feverfew, and ginseng for 2 weeks.
- Avoid ibuprofen (e.g., Advil, Motrin) and alcohol for 2 days.
- If possible, come to your appointment with a cleanly washed face.

After Treatment
- Do not massage the treated areas on the day of treatment.
- Avoid lying down for 4 hours immediately after treatment.
- Avoid applying heat to the treated area on the day of treatment.
- Avoid activities that cause facial flushing on the day of treatment, including consuming alcohol, hot tub or sauna use, exercising, and tanning.
- Gently apply a cool compress or wrapped ice pack to the treated areas for 15 minutes every few hours as needed to reduce discomfort, swelling, or bruising up to a few days after treatment. If bruising occurs, it typically resolves within 7–10 days.
- After treatment, oral consumption and/or topical application of *Arnica montana* may help to reduce bruising and swelling.
- Botulinum toxin treatment effects take about 1–2 weeks to fully develop and last approximately 2.5–4 months.
- If 1–2 weeks after treatment you feel that you require a touch-up, please contact the office.

3B. Botulinum Toxin Treatment of Underarm Sweating

Before Treatment
- Avoid aspirin (e.g., Excedrin), vitamin E, St. John's wort, and other dietary supplements including ginkgo, evening primrose oil, garlic, feverfew, and ginseng for 2 weeks.
- Avoid ibuprofen (e.g., Advil, Motrin) and alcohol for 2 days.
- Shave underarms and do not use over-the-counter deodorants or antiperspirants for 24 hours before your appointment.

After Treatment
- You may have temporary purple discoloration of the skin after treatment (because of the iodine-starch test), which will wash off over 1–2 days with regular showering/bathing.
- Do not massage the treated areas on the day of treatment.
- Avoid applying heat to the treated area on the day of treatment.
- Avoid activities that cause flushing on the day of treatment, including hot tub or sauna use, exercising, and tanning.
- Gently apply a cool compress or wrapped ice pack to the treated areas for 15 minutes every few hours as needed to reduce discomfort, swelling, or bruising up to a few days after treatment. If bruising occurs, it typically resolves within 7–10 days.
- After treatment, oral consumption and/or topical application of *Arnica montana* may help to reduce bruising and swelling.
- Botulinum toxin treatment effects take about 1–2 weeks to fully develop and last approximately 6 months.
- If 2 weeks after treatment you feel that you require a touch-up, please contact the office.

Consent Forms

4A. Botulinum Toxin Treatment of the Face and Neck

This consent form is designed to provide the information necessary when considering whether or not to undergo botulinum toxin treatment for facial and neck wrinkles with Botox®.

Injection of botulinum toxin (Botox) causes weakness of targeted muscles, which can last approximately 3–4 months. Injection of small amounts of Botox relaxes the treated muscles and can reduce facial wrinkles such as frown lines. Botox solution is injected with a small needle into the targeted muscles. Effects are typically seen in a few days and can take 1–2 weeks to fully develop.

Botox is approved by the Food and Drug Administration for the temporary treatment of moderate to severe dynamic frown lines in adults aged 18–65 years and is used off-label for all other cosmetic treatment areas.

The risks, side effects, and complications in treatment with Botox on facial and neck areas include, but are not limited to the following:

- Localized burning or stinging pain during injection
- Bruising
- Redness
- Tenderness
- Swelling
- Infection
- Numbness or dysesthesia
- Headache
- Anxiety
- Vasovagal episode with loss of consciousness
- Facial asymmetry, alteration, or poor aesthetic results
- Inadequate reduction of wrinkles or lack of intended effect
- Blepharoptosis (droopy eyelid)
- Eyebrow ptosis (droopy eyebrow)
- Photophobia (light sensitivity)
- Impaired eyelid closure and blink reflex
- Ectropian (lower eyelid exposure)
- Lagophthalmos (incomplete eyelid closure)
- Xerophthalmia (dry eyes)
- Epiphora (tearing)
- Diplopia (double vision) or vision changes
- Eye trauma
- Worsening eye bags
- Lip ptosis with resultant smile asymmetry

- Oral incompetence with resultant drooling and/or impaired speaking, eating, or drinking
- Cheek flaccidity
- Dysarthria (difficulty articulating)
- Dysphagia (difficulty swallowing), necessitating nasogastric tube placement in severe cases
- Hoarseness
- Neck weakness
- Weakening of muscles adjacent to the intended treatment area
- Autoantibodies against botulinum toxin may be present or develop after treatments rendering treatments ineffective (1–2% of patients treated for cosmetic indications per Allergan).
- Extremely rare, immediate hypersensitivity reaction with signs of urticaria, edema, and a remote possibility of anaphylaxis.
- Case reports of side effects due to distant spread from the site of injection have been reported with large doses of botulinum toxin, including generalized muscle weakness, ptosis, dysphagia, dysarthria, urinary incontinence, respiratory difficulties, and death due to respiratory compromise.

Postmarketing safety data suggest that botulinum toxin effects may, in some cases, be observed beyond the site of local injection. The symptoms may include generalized muscle weakness, double vision, blurred vision, eyelid droop, difficulty swallowing, difficulty speaking, urinary incontinence, and breathing difficulties. These symptoms have been reported hours to weeks after injection. Swallowing and breathing difficulties can be life threatening and there have been reports of death related to spread of toxin effects. The risk of symptoms is probably greatest in children treated for spasticity but symptoms can also occur in adults, particularly in those patients who have underlying conditions that would predispose them to these symptoms. No definite serious adverse event reports of distant spread of toxin effect associated with dermatologic use of cosmetic botulinum toxin at the labeled dose of 20 units (for frown lines) or 100 units (for underarm sweating) have been reported.

My signature below certifies that I have fully read this consent form and understand the information provided to me regarding the proposed procedure. I have been adequately informed about the procedure including the potential benefits, limitations, and alternative treatments, and I have had all questions and concerns answered to my satisfaction. I understand that results are not guaranteed and I accept the risks, side effects, and possible complications inherent in undergoing Botox treatments.

Patient Name _____

Patient Signature _____   Date _____

4B. Botulinum Toxin Treatment of Underarm Sweating (Axillary Hyperhidrosis)

This consent form is designed to provide the information necessary when considering whether or not to undergo botulinum toxin treatment for underarm sweating, also called primary axillary hyperhidrosis, with Botox®.

Botulinum toxin (Botox) injections can reduce underarm sweating that is not due to an underlying medical condition. Botox is approved by the Food and Drug Administration for the temporary treatment of primary axillary hyperhidrosis. Botox solution is injected with a small needle into the skin to target the sweat glands. Reduced underarm sweating is typically reported 1–2 weeks after treatment and effects last for approximately 6 months or more in some cases.

Before receiving Botox treatment for underarm sweating, you should receive an evaluation from you regular physician to ensure that you do not have an underlying medical condition that is causing the excessive underarm sweating. Also, Botox is not intended as the first treatment to prevent underarm sweating. It is indicated once other therapies such as over-the-counter antiperspirants and aluminum chloride topical antiperspirants have been tried and found ineffective.

The risks, side effects, and complications in treatment with Botox on underarm areas include, but are not limited to the following:

- Localized burning or stinging pain during injection
- Bruising
- Redness
- Tenderness
- Swelling
- Infection
- Numbness or dysesthesia
- Anxiety
- Vasovagal episode with loss of consciousness
- Inadequate reduction of sweating or lack of intended effect
- Autoantibodies against botulinum toxin may be present or develop after treatments rendering treatments ineffective (1–2% of patients treated for cosmetic indications per Allergan).
- Extremely rare, immediate hypersensitivity reaction with signs of urticaria, edema, and a remote possibility of anaphylaxis.
- Case reports of side effects due to distant spread from the site of injection have been reported with large doses of botulinum toxin, including generalized muscle weakness, ptosis, dysphagia, dysarthria, urinary incontinence, respiratory difficulties, and death due to respiratory compromise.

Postmarketing safety data suggest that botulinum toxin effects may, in some cases, be observed beyond the site of local injection. The symptoms may include generalized muscle weakness, double vision, blurred vision, eyelid droop, difficulty swallowing, difficulty speaking, urinary incontinence, and breathing difficulties. These symptoms have been reported hours to weeks after injection. Swallowing and breathing difficulties can be life threatening and there have been reports of death related to spread of toxin effects. The risk of symptoms is probably greatest in children treated for spasticity but symptoms can also occur in adults, particularly in those patients who have underlying conditions that would predispose them to these symptoms. No definite serious adverse event reports of distant spread of toxin effect associated with dermatologic use of cosmetic botulinum toxin at the labeled dose of 100 units for underarm sweating have been reported.

My signature below certifies that I have fully read this consent form and understand the information provided to me regarding the proposed procedure. I have been adequately informed about the procedure including the potential benefits, limitations, and alternative treatments, and I have had all questions and concerns answered to my satisfaction. I understand that results are not guaranteed and I accept the risks, side effects, and possible complications inherent in undergoing Botox treatments.

Patient Name _____

Patient Signature _____   Date _____

Procedure Notes

5A. Botulinum Toxin Procedure Note for Cosmetic Treatments

Name _____   DOB: _____
      Last   First

Date:		Yes	No
Changes in Medications/Allergies?			
Pregnant or Nursing?			
Changes in health status?			

Procedure:
Botox was injected SQ/IM using a ___ gauge ___ inch needle in the following area(s) below:
Botox: lot #_____ exp._____

Area:	Area:
Vol/Units:_____	Vol/Units:_____
Area:	**Follow-up/Touch-up**
Vol/Units:_____	Area: Vol/Units:_____

A/P: Static/dynamic rhytids _____ (areas)

Notes:_____
_____
_____
_____

†See Medication and Allergy List
☐ See narrative progress notes   **Performed by:** _____

S O   S=Subjective O=Objective
☐ ☐   Frown Line/Glabella complex
☐ ☐   Forehead Lines/Frontalis muscle
☐ ☐   Crows Feet/Lateral orbicularis oculi
☐ ☐   Other:_____
☐ ☐   Other:_____
☐ ☐   Other:_____
☐ R/B/C/A of procedure discussed and all questions answered.
☐ Written pre & post tx instructions given to pt. and reviewed.
☐ Consent signed in chart.

Pre-procedure:
Prepped site with alcohol
☐ Ice for anesthesia
☐ Photos taken
Other:_____

Post-procedure:
Pt. tolerated procedure _____
Bruise noted _____
☐ Applied ice

Date:		Yes	No
Changes in Medications/Allergies?			
Pregnant or Nursing?			
Changes in health status?			

Procedure:
Botox was injected SQ/IM using a ___ gauge ___ inch needle in the following area(s) below:
Botox: lot #_____ exp._____

Area:	Area:
Vol/Units:_____	Vol/Units:_____
Area:	**Follow-up/Touch-up**
Vol/Units:_____	Area: Vol/Units:_____

A/P: Static/dynamic rhytids _____ (areas)

Notes:_____
_____
_____
_____

†See Medication and Allergy List
☐ See narrative progress notes   **Performed by:** _____

S O   S=Subjective O=Objective
☐ ☐   Frown Line/Glabella complex
☐ ☐   Forehead Lines/Frontalis muscle
☐ ☐   Crows Feet/Lateral orbicularis oculi
☐ ☐   Other:_____
☐ ☐   Other:_____
☐ ☐   Other:_____
☐ R/B/C/A of procedure discussed and all questions answered.
☐ Written pre & post tx instructions given to pt. and reviewed.
☐ Consent signed in chart.

Preprocedure:
Prepped site with alcohol
☐ Ice for anesthesia
☐ Photos taken
Other:_____

Postprocedure:
Pt. tolerated procedure _____
Bruise noted _____
☐ Applied ice

5B. Botulinum Toxin Treatment Note for Axillary Hyperhidrosis

Name: _____ D.O.B.: _____ Date: _____
       Last   First

History of Present Illness: _____

_____

Prior treatments:_____

- Over-the-counter antiperspirants used with inadequate response.
- Drysol (aluminum chloride) used with inadequate response.

Hyperhidrosis Severity Scale:
1. (unnoticeable) = My underarm sweating is never noticeable and never interferes with my daily activities.
2. (tolerable) = My underarm sweating is sometimes noticeable and sometimes interferes with my daily activities.
3. (barely tolerable) = My underarm sweating is frequently noticeable and frequently interferes with daily activities.
4. (intolerable) = My underarm sweating is always noticeable and always interferes with my daily activities.
   - Do you change shirts during the day because of excessive sweating? Y ☐ N ☐
   - Other areas of excessive sweating: _____

Diagnosis: Primary axillary hyperhidrosis.

Minor's Iodine-Starch Test:

The patient's underarm area was shaved. Iodine solution was applied to each axilla and allowed to dry fully. Corn starch was sprinkled on the treatment areas and extra starch brushed off. Ten minutes after application, the axillae skin turned deep blue-black color in the areas of greatest perspiration. A surgical marking pen was used to draw a line around the perspiration treatment area.

Botox treatment:

Botox was reconstituted as follows: 100 units of Botox in 4.0-mL 0.9% nonpreserved saline. The treatment area was cleansed with alcohol and injection points marked with a marking pen. Injections were placed intradermally with 0.1 mL of Botox (2.5 units) at each site for a total of _____ units with _____ injections in the right axilla and _____ units with _____ injections in the left axilla, using a 30-gauge 0.5-inch needle. Injections were spaced 1–2 cm apart, within the area of perspiration.

_____

_____

Complications: None/_____ **Blood loss:** <1 mL/_____

Condition on leaving: _____

Performed by: _____

Supply Sources

Botulinum Toxin

Allergan, Inc.
Botox®
Phone: 1-800-377-7790
www.allergan.com

Medicis Pharmaceutical Corporation
Dysport®
Phone: 602-808-8800
www.medicis.com

Topical Anesthetics

American Health Solutions Pharmacy
Benzocaine/lidocaine/tetracaine (BLT) (20:6:4) ointment
1-310-838-7422.
www.AHSRx.com

APP Pharmaceuticals
EMLA® (lidocaine 2.5% : prilocaine 2.5%)
Schaumburg, IL 60173-5837
1-847-413-2075
www.apppharma.com

PharmaDerm
L-M-X® (lidocaine 4%–5%)
1-973-514-4240
www.pharmaderm.com

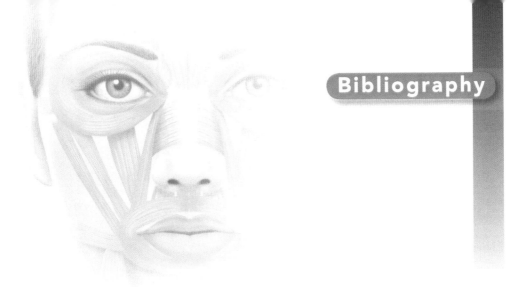

General

Carruthers J, Fagien S, Matarasso SL, et al. The Botox consensus group: Consensus recommendations on the use of botulinum toxin type A in facial aesthetics. Plas Recon Surg. 2004;114(6)(supp):1S–22S.

Small R. Aesthetic procedures in office practice. Am Fam Physician. 2009;80(11):1231–1237.

Small R. Botulinum Toxin. In: Usatine R, Pfenninger J, Stuhlberg D, and Small R, eds. Dermatologic and Cosmetic Procedures in Office Practice. Philadelphia, PA. Elsevier. Pending 2011.

Small R. Botulinum Toxin Type A for Facial Rejuvenation. In: Mayeaux E, ed. The Essential Guide to Primary Care Procedures. Philadelphia, PA. Lippincott Williams & Wilkins. 2009:200–213.

Small R. Aesthetic Principles and Consultation. In: Usatine R, Pfenninger J, Stuhlberg D, and Small R, eds. Dermatologic and Cosmetic Procedures in Office Practice. Philadelphia, PA. Elsevier. Pending 2011.

Small R. Aesthetic Procedures Introduction. In: Mayeaux E, ed. The Essential Guide to Primary Care Procedures. Philadelphia, PA. Lippincott Williams & Wilkins. 2009:195–199.

Small R and Hoang D. Combining Cosmetic Treatments. In: Usatine R, Pfenninger J, Stuhlberg D, and Small R, eds. Dermatologic and Cosmetic Procedures in Office Practice. Philadelphia, PA. Elsevier. Pending 2011.

Sommer B, Zschocke I, Bergfeld D, et al. Satisfaction of patients after treatment with botulinum toxin for dynamic facial lines. Derm Surg. 2003;29:456.

Reconstitution

Alam M, Dover JS, Arndt KA. Pain associated with injection of botulinum A exotoxin reconstituted using isotonic sodium chloride with and without preservative: a double-blind, randomized controlled trial. Arch Dermatol. 2002;138(4):510–514.

Carruthers A, Carruthers J, Cohen J. Dilution volume of botulinum toxin type A for the treatment of glabellar rhytides: does it matter? Derm Surg. 2007;33:S97–S104.

Hexsel DM, De Almeida AT, Rutowitsch M, et al. Multicenter double-blind study of the efficacy of injections with botulinum toxin type A reconstituted up to 6 weeks before application. Derm Surg. 2003;29:523.

Aftercare

Hsu TS, Dover JS, Kaminer MS, et al. Why make patients exercise facial muscles for 4 hours after botulinum toxin treatment? Arch Dermatol. 2003;139(7):948.

Complications

Carruthers A, Bogle M, Carruthers J, et al. A randomized, evaluator-blinded, two-center study of the safety and effect of volume on the diffusion and efficacy of botulinum toxin type A in the treatment of lateral orbital rhytides. Derm Surg. 2007;33(5):567–571.

Carruthers A, Carruthers J. Clinical indications and injection techniques for the cosmetic use of botulinum A exotoxin. Derm Surg. 1998;24:1189–1194.

Carruthers J, Lowe NJ, Menter MA, et al. A multicenter, double-blind, randomized, placebo-controlled study of the efficacy and safety of botulinum toxin type A in the treatment of glabellar lines. J Am Acad Dermatol. 2002;46(6):840–849.

Fagien S. Temporary management of upper lid ptosis, lid malposition, and eyelid fissure asymmetry with botulinum toxin type A. Plast Reconstr Surg. 2004;114(7):1892–1902.

Klein AW. Complications, adverse reactions, and insights with the use of botulinum toxin. Derm Surg. 2003;29:549–556.

Klein AW. Complications and adverse reactions with the use of botulinum toxin. Dis Mon. 2002;48:336–356.

Klein AW. Contraindications and complications with the use of botulinum toxin. Clin Dermatol. 2004;22(1):66–75.

Upper Face

Carruthers J, Carruthers A. The use of botulinum toxin type A in the upper face. Facial Plast Surg Clin North Am. 2006;14(3):253–260.

Maas CS. Botulinum neurotoxins and injectable fillers: minimally invasive management of the aging upper face. Facial Plast Surg Clin North Am. 2006;14(3):241–245.

Frown Lines

Carruthers J, Lowe NJ, Menter MA, et al. A multicenter, double-blind, randomized, placebo-controlled study of the efficacy and safety of botulinum toxin type A in the treatment of glabellar lines. J Am Acad Dermatol. 2002;46(6):840–849.

Carruthers J, Lowe NJ, Menter MA, et al. Double-blind, placebo-controlled study of the safety and efficacy of botulinum toxin type A for patients with glabellar lines. Plast Reconstr Surg. 2003;112(4):1089–1098.

Horizontal Forehead Lines

Carruthers A, Carruthers J, Cohen JL. A prospective, double-blind, randomized, parallel- group, dose-ranging study of botulinum toxin type A in female subjects with horizontal forehead rhytides. Derm Surg. 2003;29(5): 461–467.

Crow's Feet

Balikian RV, Zimbler MS. Primary and adjunctive uses of botulinum toxin type A in the periorbital region. Otolaryngol Clin North Am. 2007;40(2):291–303.

Lowe NJ, Lask GP, Yamauchi PS, et al. Bilateral, double-blind, randomized comparison of 3 doses of botulinum toxin type A and placebo in patients with crow's feet. J Am Acad Dermatol. 2002;47(6):834–840.

Lower Eyelid Wrinkles

Flynn TC, Carruthers A, Carruthers J. Botulinum-A toxin treatment of the lower eyelid improves infraorbital rhytides and widens the eye. Dermatol Surg. 2001;27(8):703–708.

Flynn TC, Carruthers J, Carruthers A, et al. Botulinum A toxin (BOTOX) in the lower eyelid: dose-finding study. Dermatol Surg. 2003;29(9):943–950.

Eyebrow Lift

Ahn MS, Catten M, Maas CS. Temporal brow lift using botulinum toxin A. Plas Reconstr Surg. 2000;105: 1129–1135.

Frankel AS, Kamer FM. Chemical browlift. Arch Otolaryngol Head Neck Surg. 1998;124:321–323.

Huang W, Rogachefsky AS, Foster JA. Browlift with botulinum toxin. Dermatol Surg. 2000;26(1):55–60.

Middle and Lower Face

Carruthers J, Carruthers A. Botox use in the mid and lower face and neck. Semin Cutan Med Surg. 2001;20(2): 85–92.

Carruthers J, Carruthers A. Botulinum toxin A in the mid and lower face and neck. Dermatol Clin. 2004;22(2): 51–158.

Carruthers J, Carruthers A. Botulinum toxin below the eyes. Int Ophthalmol Clin. 2005;45(3):133–141.

Bunny Lines

Tamura BM, Odo MY, Chang B, et al. Treatment of nasal wrinkles with botulinum toxin. Dermatol Surg. 2005;31(3):271–275.

Lip Lines

Kaplan SE, Sherris DA, Gassner HG, et al. The use of botulinum toxin A in perioral rejuvenation. Facial Plast Surg Clin North Am. 2007;15(4):415–421, v–vi.

Gummy Smile

Polo M. Botulinum toxin type A (Botox) for the neuromuscular correction of excessive gingival display on smiling (gummy smile). Am J Orthod Dentofacial Orthop. 2008;133(2):195–203.

Marionette Lines

Gassia V, Beylot C, Bechaux S, et al. Botulinum toxin injection techniques in the lower third and middle of the face, the neck, and the decollete: the "Nefertiti lift." [in French]. Ann Dermatol Venereol. 2009;136(suppl 4):S111–S118.

Chin

Papel ID, Capone RB. Botulinum toxin A for mentalis muscle dysfunction. Arch Facial Plast Surg. 2001;3(4): 268–269.

Neck Bands

Brandt FS, Boker A. Botulinum toxin for the treatment of neck lines and neck bands. Dermatol Clin. 2004;22: 159–166.
Matarasso A, Matarasso SL, Brandt FS, et al. Botulinum A exotoxin for the management of platysma bands. Plast Reconstr Surg. 1999;103(2):645–652.

Axillary Hyperhidrosis

Absar MS, Onwudike M. Efficacy of botulinum toxin type A in the treatment of focal axillary hyperhidrosis. Dermatol Surg. 2008;34(6):751–755.
Hornberger J, Grimes K, Naumann M, et al. Recognition, diagnosis, and treatment of primary focal hyperhidrosis. J Am Acad Dermatol. 2004;51(2):274–286.
Kowalski JW, Eadie N, Daggett S. Development, validity, and reliability of the Hyperhidrosis Disease Severity Scale (HDSS). Poster Presented at: 62nd Annual Meeting of the American Academy of Dermatology; February 6–10, 2004; Washington, DC.
Lowe NJ, Glaser DA, Eadie N, et al. Botulinum toxin type A in the treatment of primary axillary hyperhidrosis: a 52-week multicenter double-blind, randomized, placebo-controlled study of efficacy and safety. J Am Acad Dermatol. 2007;56(4):604–611.
Strutton DS, Kowalski JW, Glaser DA, et al. US prevalence of hyperhidrosis and impact on individuals with axillary hyperhidrosis: results from a national survey. J Am Acad Dermatol. 2004;51(2):241–248.

Combining Aesthetic Treatments

Blitzer A, Binder WJ, Boyd J, et al, eds. Management of Facial Lines and Wrinkles. Philadelphia, PA. Lippincott Williams & Wilkins. 2000.
Carruthers J, Carruthers A. A prospective, randomized, parallel group study analyzing the effect of BTX-A (Botox) and nonanimal sourced hyaluronic acid (NASHA, Restylane) in combination compared with NASHA (Restylane) alone in severe glabellar rhytides in adult female subjects: treatment of severe glabellar rhytides with a hyaluronic acid derivative compared with the derivative and BTX-A. Derm Surg. 2003;29(8):802–809.
Carruthers J, Glogau RG, Blitzer A. Advances in facial rejuvenation: botulinum toxin type A, hyaluronic acid dermal fillers, and combination therapies—consensus recommendations. Plast Reconstr Surg. 2008;121(suppl 5): 5S–30S.
Coleman KR, Carruthers J. Combination therapy with BOTOX and fillers: the new rejuvenation paradigm. Dermatol Ther. 2006;19(3):177–188.
De Maio M. Botulinum toxin in association with other rejuvenation methods. J Cosmet Laser Ther. 2003;5(3–4): 210–212.
De Maio M. Combination Therapy—The Microlift Procedure. In: De Maio M, Rzany B, eds. Botulinum Toxin in Aesthetic Medicine. New York, NY. Springer. 2007:127–136.
Fedok FG. Advances in minimally invasive facial rejuvenation. Curr Opin Otolaryngol Head Neck Surg. 2008;16(4):359–368.
Micheals J, Micheals B. Coupling advanced injection techniques for cosmetic enhancement. Cosmet Dermatol. 2008;21(1):31–36.

Dysport

Lowe P, Patnaik R, Lowe N. Comparison of two formulations of botulinum toxin type A for the treatment of glabellar lines: a double-blind, randomized study. J Am Acad Dermatol. 2006;55(6):975–980.

Monheit G, Carruthers A, Brandt F, et al. A randomized, double-blind, placebo-controlled study of botulinum toxin type-A for the treatment of glabellar line: determination of optimal dose. Derm Surg. 2007;33(suppl 1): S51–S59.

Moy R, Maas C, Monheit G, et al. Long-term safety and efficacy of a new botulinum toxin type A in treating glabellar lines. Arch Facial Plast Surg. 2009;11(2):77–83.

Trindade De Almeda AR, Marques E, de Almeida J, et al. Pilot study comparing the diffusion of two formulations of botulinum toxin type A in patients with forehead hyperhydrosis. Derm Surg. 2007;33:S37–S43.

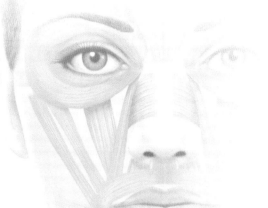

Note: Page numbers followed by f and t indicates figure and table respectively.